W9-AZZ-629

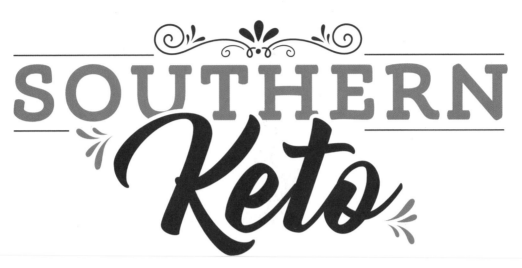

SOUTHERN Keto

100+ Traditional Food Favorites for a Low-Carb Lifestyle

Natasha Newton

VICTORY BELT PUBLISHING

Las Vegas

I dedicate this book to my beloved Southern grandmas, Ida Mae and Isabell—not only because they were great Southern cooks, but also because they lived a life of kindness and grace and in service to others. They both embodied what it means to be a Proverbs 31 woman. I hope to carry on their legacy of light and love.

First Published in 2019 by Victory Belt Publishing Inc.

Copyright © 2019 Natasha Newton

All rights reserved

No part of this publication may be reproduced or distributed in any form or by any means, electronic or mechanical, or stored in a database or retrieval system, without prior written permission from the publisher.

ISBN-13: 978-1-628603-13-2

The author is not licensed a practitioner, physician, or medical professional and offers no medical diagnoses, treatments, suggestions, or counseling. The information presented herein has not been evaluated by the U.S. Food and Drug Administration, and it is not intended to diagnose, treat, cure, or prevent any disease. Full medical clearance from a licensed physician should be obtained before beginning or modifying any diet, exercise, or lifestyle program, and physicians should be informed of all nutritional changes.

The author/owner claims no responsibility to any person or entity for any liability, loss, or damage caused or alleged to be caused directly or indirectly as a result of the use, application, or interpretation of the information presented herein.

Front and back cover photos and Fruit Pizza photo by Hayley Mason and Bill Staley

Cover design by Justin-Aaron Velasco

Interior design by Yordan Terziev and Boryana Yordanova

Printed in Canada

TC 0519

❧ Contents ❧

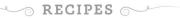

RECIPES

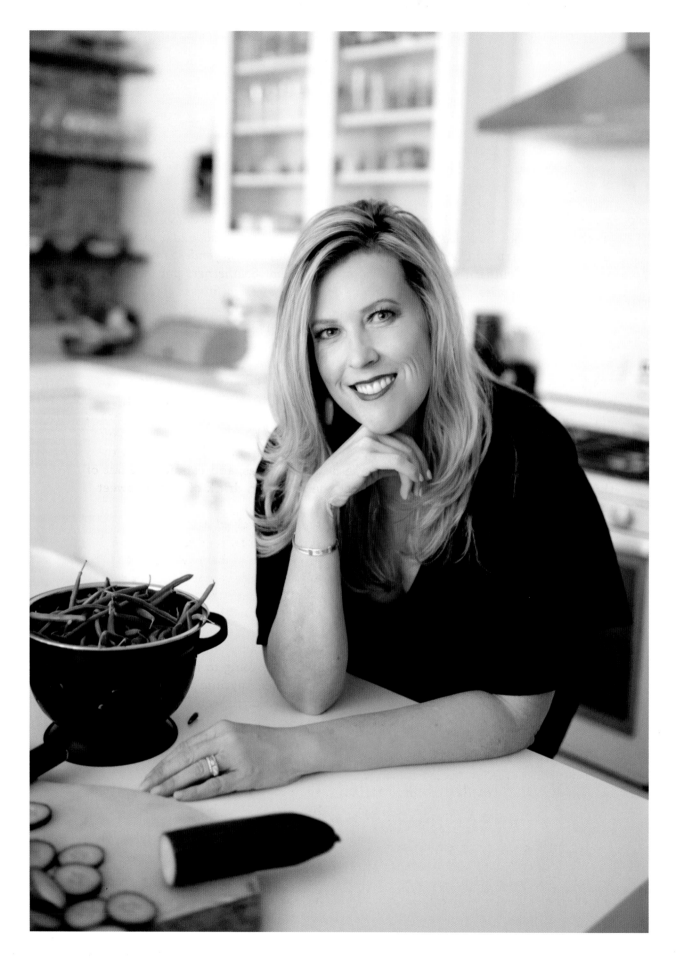

Southern Heritage

Hey y'all! Come on in, take your shoes off, and stay awhile! Can I get you anything to eat or drink? Yes, this is the way most conversations began when a guest entered my childhood home. Southern hospitality is still alive and well. We are proud to carry on the traditions of our grandmothers. My fondest memories of growing up Southern involve the love and effort that Southerners put into their food. These memories are ingrained in my heart and my soul forever.

I grew up in south-central Kentucky, and I've lived in Tennessee for the past twenty years. Depending on which part of the South you are from, the cuisine is likely to vary. Traditional Southern foods are known to be breaded and deep-fried, most likely in bacon drippings or lard like our grandmas used. Lots of fresh garden-grown vegetables can always be found. In addition to beef and pork, wild game meat such as venison, squirrel, rabbit, and turkey are plentiful. If you are lucky enough to live in the Southern coastal regions, you also have access to fresh fish, crab, oysters, and shrimp. Food and drink are central to our Southern roots. The rich homemade desserts, cakes, and candies are out of this world! And of course, we can't forget the Southern drink of choice, sweet tea!

Growing up, I remember every family gathering revolved around the fabulous food our mommas and grandmas would prepare. It was made with love, and lots of it! Where I'm from, when someone has a baby, we take the family a meal. If someone is ill or has had surgery, we take the family a meal. If someone loses a loved one, we take food to the family during their time of mourning. It's an act of love that we take very seriously. We wouldn't have it any other way.

You've probably heard the phrase "Southern hospitality" many times. If you visit us, we want you to feel right at home, and we're going to feed you! That's how I was raised. I get it from my Grandma Ida Mae. Anytime we would go to her house, she would feed us. Even if you didn't think you were hungry, you would want to find something to eat at Grandma's house. Later, after I got married and my husband and I would visit, she would say to me, "Fix your husband something to eat." He always got a kick out of that! Being of an older generation, she also expected me to wait on my husband.

When I eat foods like the ones she used to prepare, I am instantly transported back in time. Life was simpler then. It was all about the love of family and friends gathered together for the holidays, special occasions, and church potlucks. In my experience, that's why comfort food is called just that. No matter what area or culture we grow up in, we associate food with comfort and our memories of time spent with loved ones. It is very important to me to keep those traditions alive no matter which way of eating we choose.

In this book, I'm sharing mostly iconic dishes from my childhood. I've worked to convert Southern comfort foods like Grandma used to make to fit a low-carb, ketogenic lifestyle. The recipes in this book are not going to taste *exactly* like your grandmother's food. Let's face it, no one can compete with that! But we can get pretty darn close. If Ida Mae were still alive, I'm not sure she would agree with the culinary changes I've made to these traditional Southern dishes, but I do believe she would be proud! Throughout my childhood, she worried a lot about my weight and health. I know it would make her happy to see me so much stronger and healthier.

Grandma would start preparing holiday meals weeks in advance. She put so much love into the food she made for our family. I, too, love cooking holiday meals; there's something special about planning and preparing meals that I know my family will love. I have successfully prepared ketogenic meals for birthdays, Thanksgiving, and even Christmas! I truly believe it is possible to stay on track and not feel deprived on such occasions. And avoiding those feelings of guilt that come from overindulging in foods that aren't good for you is great.

When I got married, I didn't know how to cook much besides spaghetti. I know you're thinking, *Wait a minute, didn't your grandma teach you how to cook?* I was definitely influenced by watching Ida Mae cook for years, but I didn't take the time to learn for myself until I was older. I taught myself to cook by following recipes in old church fundraiser cookbooks and in *Southern Living* magazine, which I received monthly. I was fortunate to live up the road from my grandparents and watched my grandma cook so many times. I believe that's why cooking comes naturally to me. Of course, I was drawn to Southern comfort food and lots of carbs! Once I became comfortable and confident in my ketogenic cooking skills, I became interested in remaking all the comfort foods that my family loves low-carb. I've found that many of my old family recipes can be converted to keto recipes.

There's a learning curve to ketogenic cooking and baking, but once you get the basics down, you'll find yourself wanting to "keto-fy" everything. With this cookbook, I hope to help you think outside the box when it comes to keeping ketogenic food interesting, no matter the type of cuisine you choose. Making it fun is how I have been able to sustain this lifestyle long term!

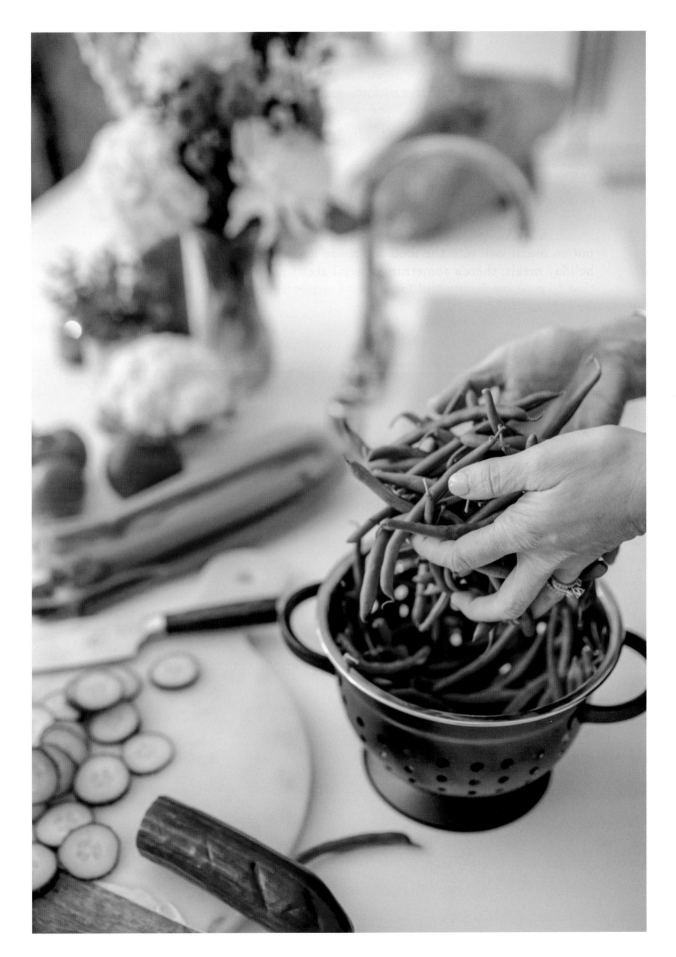

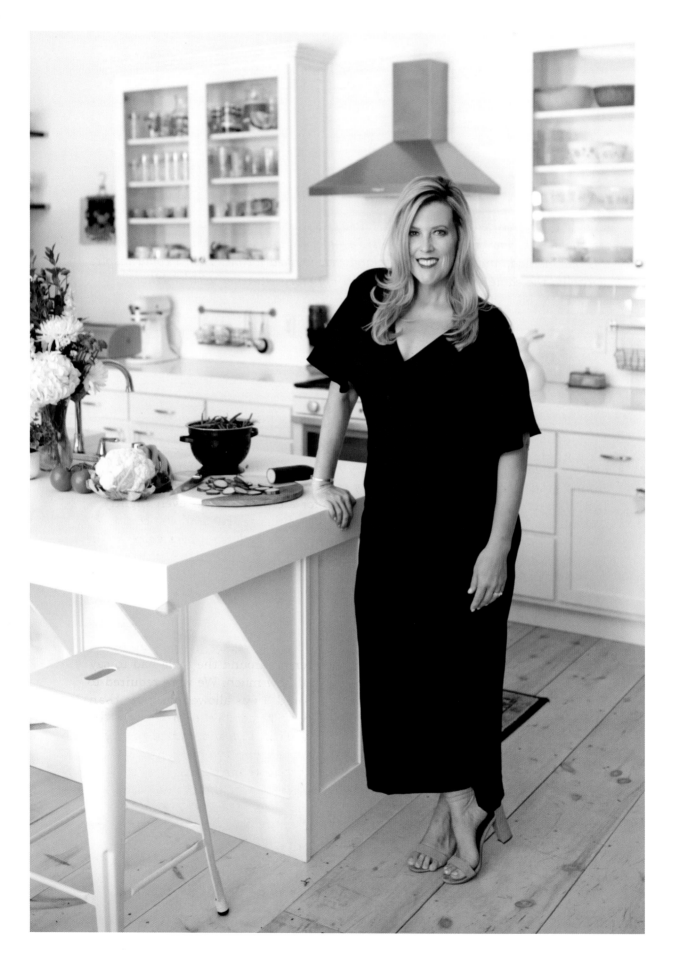

⧽ My Story ⧼

Mine is a complicated and somewhat messy story. I wish I had a definitive testimonial for you that went like this: I was obese and lost all this weight using this one method, and that's the one thing that worked for me. Then I could inspire you to do the same. Instead, I will tell you my story, starting with childhood obesity and how it affected me in my adult years. I do hope it inspires you. I want you to know that despite failing what seemed like hundreds of times, I finally found what works for me. I encourage you to never give up. Never stop searching for what works for you. You can have success and live the life you desire. I truly believe that if I can do it, anyone can!

Struggling with my weight growing up

From a very young age, I didn't really feel like I fit in with other kids. I had a wonderful loving family, and they didn't treat me any differently, but around grade-school age, I became very self-aware of my body image. In the 1980s, there weren't many clothing options for a child who was even slightly overweight. My mom bought me mostly dresses because that's all she could find to fit my shape, aside from boys' husky-size jeans. I remember being a Girl Scout and so wanting to dress like the other scouts. They all matched in their uniforms with pants, while mine was of course a Girl Scout dress, but we were happy that there was a dress option! That was only the beginning of my desire to fit in and be what I considered normal.

I was placed on my first real diet at the age of nine. It was a medically supervised diet at a local doctor's office and involved a weekly group meeting with all adults. We would weigh in, and then each person around the table had to say whether he or she had lost or gained weight and how much. We were required to keep a weekly food journal, and it was calorie based. I was allowed no more than 1,200 calories and 20 grams of fat per day. I don't remember losing any weight on that program. I was only nine; my heart wasn't in it! I just wanted to be like other nine-year-olds, who only had to think about playing and other fun things. I want to make it clear that I do not blame my parents for putting me in this program! They were just concerned parents doing the best they could for their overweight child. Being a parent myself has helped me understand that even more. They were worried about my health, and I'm thankful they tried. No one else in our family was overweight, so they didn't know how to deal with it.

I've struggled with my weight for as long as I can remember. I always had an unhealthy obsession with food. My mom wouldn't keep much junk food at home because she worried that I would eat it all. As soon as I left her sight

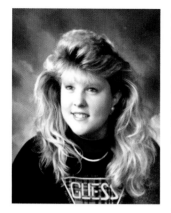

and got to family and friends' houses, I would eat whatever I could get my hands on—especially sugary cereals that weren't available at my house. Sometimes to the point of making myself sick. It was the 1980s, and the fat-free diet fad was in full force! I remember eating lots of rice cakes and thinking how flavorless they were. Mom, an avid walker, would try to get me to exercise with her. She would take long walks and ask me to join her. Again, my heart wasn't in it. I would reluctantly go along but would take as many breaks as possible, always letting her walk ahead.

These early struggles set the stage for my lifelong battle with low self-esteem and food addiction. I didn't know it was food addiction. I didn't know I was addicted to sugar and carbs. After all, *fat* was the enemy, not sugar! I remember genuinely wanting to lose weight and be what I considered normal. I tried every diet imaginable, but I never followed through. The first time I lost a significant amount of weight, I was eighteen years old, and I took the prescription weight-loss pill known as fen-phen (now believed to have contributed to many deaths and illnesses). Like the many other diets I'd tried over the years, the results didn't last. I lost a lot of weight and gained it all back. My love for sugar and carbs always won out. I thought I didn't have willpower. No matter how much weight-loss success I had, I would always gain the weight back—and then some! This led to severe depression and self-loathing, not to mention the effects it had on my body, health, and relationships.

Growing up, I had good friends, and thankfully I don't remember being bullied because of my weight. In general, it was more a feeling of not belonging. My self-esteem was very low, and it held me back from participating in the extracurricular activities that other kids my age were doing. I also let it hold me back academically. I didn't try very hard, and I had no belief in myself. The teen years are hard enough without battling obesity!

I met my husband when I was twenty. When we met, I was on the lower end of my weight range after one of my many diets. We fell in love immediately and have been together ever since. He has stuck with me through all the ups and downs of my weight and health struggles. He has never once judged me or made me feel any less loved. I'm so thankful for him and his unconditional support throughout the years. No matter how much he loved me, though, I still didn't love myself, and at times that lack of self-esteem strained our relationship.

My highest known weight was 309 pounds. I was likely bigger, but at some point I stopped weighing myself. I was in denial that I had let my weight get so far out of control. One day I was reading my medical record and saw that the doctor had described me as "morbidly obese." Those words stung. I kept staring at them and reading them over and over. I thought to myself, *I'm twenty-five years old and I could die because of my weight.* You'd think that would have been the turning point, but it wasn't. I continued with yo-yo dieting, but my unhealthy obsession with food always won out. I kept searching for the next big thing—a new diet or pill that would magically fix me.

I was working in home health and a patient asked me, "When is your baby due?" Humiliation washed over me. My baby was two years old at the time! The same thing happened when I was out shopping another day. I've since learned never to ask someone when her baby is due. Just don't.

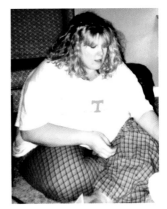

I was deeply depressed, which led to more eating and more weight gain. I was so embarrassed and avoided any and all social situations I could. One day at church, I sat down in a chair that had arms. I had sat in that chair many times before, and this time I was barely able to squeeze into it. I knew I was reaching the point of no return, and I felt like a ticking time bomb. I went on another diet and started walking. Over the next few months, I lost 50 pounds. Then I found out that I was pregnant with my second child, and I vowed to be healthier during that pregnancy. I went off the diet I'd been following, but I didn't gain too much weight.

After my son was born and I was cleared by my doctor, I began an exercise routine. I lost a lot more weight, but I wasn't eating healthfully, and I wasn't enjoying the food I was eating. In fact, I didn't eat much at all. My hair started to fall out because I was eating so poorly. At one point, my total weight loss reached around 150 pounds. I was the smallest I had ever been. The joy that came from that accomplishment was short-lived, though. In the next year, I was diagnosed with Crohn's disease. (I'll talk more about that in a bit.) The next few years were a blur of flare-ups and hospitalizations. I felt so alone and like every aspect of my life was spiraling out of control. It is thought to be common for people who have Crohn's disease to become underweight, but that wasn't the case for me; I managed to gain back all but about 50 of the pounds I had lost. As they say, old habits die hard, and once again I was finding solace in food.

Over the next several years, my struggles with food addiction and weight continued. Sometimes I felt hopeless, and food was my only comfort. It's really hard to think about it now, and even harder to openly share it with so many people. Even though I struggled with my health and weight, I was blessed with a wonderful life. I had a devoted husband and beautiful children, and here I was basing my self-worth on a number on a scale. I have so many regrets, and that is one of them. I do wish I had loved myself more throughout the process, but hindsight is always twenty-twenty.

By the age of thirty-nine, I thought I was destined to struggle with my weight forever. After giving up what seemed like hundreds of times, I decided to try something different. I was seeing things online about low-carb and keto. I knew about low-carb and had probably tried it for a day or two before, but it seemed boring and unsustainable to me. I kept seeing it pop up here and there, though, and I thought, *Why not? I've tried everything else, why not try this, too?* What really piqued my curiosity wasn't so much the weight loss; I had seen plenty of before-and-after pictures with every diet. I myself had lost huge amounts of weight on various other diets. What attracted me to keto was that people were talking about not being hungry and how eating fat kept them satisfied. After a lifetime of counting calories and fat, this blew my mind. Could it be true? Could I really eat fat, lose weight, and not be hungry while doing it? It went against everything I knew at that point.

I dove into research and read everything I could find online. I researched A LOT! When I decide to do something, I want to know *all* the details. When I felt like I had learned enough to get started, I was excited to try it. I quickly became obsessed with sugar and carbs. I was very strict in the beginning; I didn't even allow myself keto treats. I wasn't hungry and lost 20 pounds pretty fast. In my mind, this was just a diet. With that mindset, old tendencies set in, and I had my first binge. I thought, *Well, that's it. This is me; this is what I do. I sabotage every good thing that happens to me.* I felt sorry for myself for a while. I made excuses and thought, *Well, maybe the keto diet isn't for me, either.*

It took a few weeks, but I had this nagging feeling that I was missing out on something big. I had learned too much about keto to just forget everything. I decided to try again. This time I went in with a different mindset. My usual all-or-nothing approach wasn't going to get me very far; I was finally realizing that it only increases my tendency to binge. This time, I would allow myself more grace. I had to start viewing it as a lifestyle change. This was not easy for me, and I fell off the wagon a few more times, but then something clicked, and I found myself not wanting to go back to my old ways. Every part of me was being renewed. It wasn't just the weight I was losing. My mind felt clearer than ever before. This is where the "keto is life" philosophy comes in. One day I was feeling so positive about the changes I was experiencing from the inside out that I thought to myself, *Keto is life!* It wasn't just a fad diet to me; I had tried all those. This one was life-changing. My life was changing. For the first time, I felt like I was in control.

I threw myself into making keto more sustainable and less boring, and I continued making changes to my lifestyle. I stopped relying on the scale to make me feel successful. I focused more on how my clothes fit and the smaller sizes I could wear. I reached what I felt was a good point and was able to maintain it. Maintaining a lower weight was something I had never been able to do before.

I realize now that eating a lot of sugar was holding me back. The more sugar I ate, the more I wanted. Living a ketogenic lifestyle is the only thing I've ever tried that actually helped with my food and sugar addiction. Keto keeps me feeling full and satiated and keeps my blood glucose stable; therefore, I don't have the intense sugar cravings that I used to.

I was obsessed with food. It's embarrassing to admit, but it's true. I hope that admitting it will help others who are dealing with the same shame to admit it, too. In my opinion, there isn't a lot of support out there for food addiction. People who are addicted to food are sometimes viewed as lazy and lacking in self-discipline. I know that every individual is different and that the same treatment will not work for everyone, but I am passionate about sharing what worked for me. After spending decades on the dieting roller coaster, I truly believe that if I can change, anyone can. My hope is that you don't wait as long as I did to find your answer. Getting started is the hardest part, but if you commit, it will get easier!

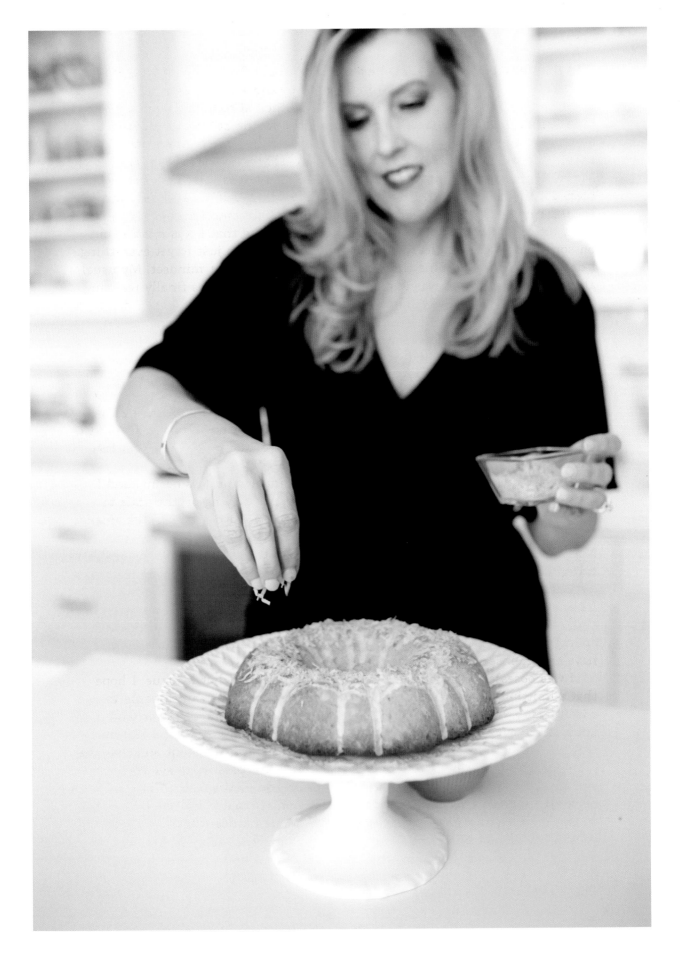

Living with Crohn's disease

NOTE: This is my own personal experience and is not intended to be taken as medical advice.

I was diagnosed with moderate to severe Crohn's disease in 2004, at the age of twenty-nine. With that diagnosis, my life and my young family's life were turned upside down. Until that time, I was seemingly healthy, other than my weight. I had two young children to care for, ages eighteen months and five years. Some of those years are a blur. It was a painful time in my life, and it's still hard to think and talk about. My illness strained my family emotionally and financially. I was constantly in and out of the hospital. To this day, I still sometimes struggle with the guilt I feel over missing so much of my kids' lives when they were young. My faith, my family, and a few close friends are what got me through those hard times.

For about a year, I did everything I could to avoid biologic drugs. I was scared to death to take Remicade infusions because I had read a lot about them and knew that they came with risks. I tried every natural remedy and every piece of nutritional advice people threw at me. It wasn't working; I kept getting sicker and sicker. I wanted so badly to be well for my kids and husband, so finally I gave in. I had to try something more because I was at the end of my resources, and I was desperate for any possible relief. On most days I felt like I was dying, and I couldn't function well enough to take care of my kids. We didn't have family nearby. At that time, not many other medications had been developed for Crohn's disease.

The Remicade did help, but not immediately. I would say the improvement was very gradual; I could function and take care of basic responsibilities again, but something was still missing. Over the years I kept looking for ways to feel better—some magic vitamin or supplement that would help. Trust me, people were always giving me advice, even when I didn't ask for it. I tried every new thing that came along. I struggled with fatigue, sometimes severe. My doctors didn't have answers for me and would say that the Remicade was working and keeping me in remission—*their* definition of remission. But I didn't have full quality of life. Given how good I feel now, I know that I had a lot of inflammation in my body back then.

In 2013, I had colon resection surgery. My diseased colon had so much scar tissue built up that it had become a dangerous risk for complete obstruction. I'd known the surgery was a possibility since I was first diagnosed, and the thought of it scared me to death. The doctors removed 1 foot of my small intestine and 2 feet of my large intestine. I didn't have to have a colostomy, but I knew it could happen with a surgery like that. I required another major surgery in 2015 to correct complications that had developed from the colon resection. That was during the time I was really getting into the ketogenic lifestyle.

The big question people ask me a lot is, has keto helped your Crohn's disease? Let me start by saying that I did not start keto to help with my Crohn's disease. Truly, my reason for starting keto was just to lose weight. Even with Crohn's disease, I was still overweight. But to my surprise, I found that after committing to keto for an extended period, my health has benefited in ways I hadn't imagined. I feel stronger and my mind feels clearer. Keto hasn't "cured" the Crohn's disease, but I feel better than I have in years!

Yes, I still take the infusions. At this point in my life, I'm not willing to risk stopping them because Remicade is the only medicine that has given me any relief. I was told that it sometimes stops working for people after a few years and that it normally doesn't work for as long as it has for me. Before keto, and even after I started taking Remicade, I still struggled with inflammation and fatigue. Crohn's is an autoimmune disease, and inflammation is my body's way of fighting. I've had to follow my heart and do what I feel is right for me. The ketogenic lifestyle has improved my overall sense of well-being. Now, I have more good days than bad, and I don't have the extreme fatigue that I used to suffer from. Oh, yes, occasionally I still have a bad day, but I can usually connect that to stress or just being overly busy.

My family and friends have noticed the positive changes in me as well. They comment on how much better I look and seem to feel. I have been offered antidepressants a few times, but I never took them. I'm not knocking them— they have their place—but I told the doctor that I knew why I was depressed: because I was sick all the time! I applaud people who never have to take medicine for their autoimmune disease and have healed their bodies with food alone. Having an autoimmune disease is terrible and complicated because no two people are alike. I would never judge anyone else's path to wellness. I say this because I don't want people who need to take medicine to feel bad because others are having success without it. This goes back to doing what works for you. Medicine and nutrition together are giving me a better quality of life. Having an autoimmune disease took its toll on my emotional health over the years, but the ketogenic lifestyle has helped me feel better mentally, too, and for that I am grateful!

Getting Started with Keto

The ketogenic diet is a low-carbohydrate, moderate-protein, high-fat way of eating. Most people on keto eat 20 to 50 grams of net carbs per day. When fed this way, the body produces ketones to use for energy rather than relying on glucose.

Before you start keto, I recommend that you do your own research. Knowledge is power. Keto isn't one-size-fits-all, and one person doesn't have all the answers. In the Resources section on page 286, I recommend a few books and websites that can help you learn more.

Figuring net carbs

On a ketogenic diet, it is common to count net carbs rather than total carbs based on the idea that certain carbohydrates like fiber and sugar alcohols do not increase blood glucose levels. Here's how you calculate net carbs:

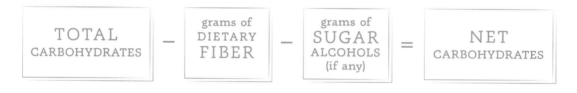

TOTAL CARBOHYDRATES − grams of DIETARY FIBER − grams of SUGAR ALCOHOLS (if any) = NET CARBOHYDRATES

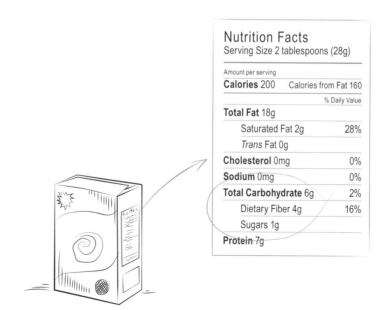

Nutrition Facts		
Serving Size 2 tablespoons (28g)		
Amount per serving		
Calories 200	Calories from Fat 160	
		% Daily Value
Total Fat 18g		
Saturated Fat 2g		28%
Trans Fat 0g		
Cholesterol 0mg		0%
Sodium 0mg		0%
Total Carbohydrate 6g		2%
Dietary Fiber 4g		16%
Sugars 1g		
Protein 7g		

Counting macros versus intuitive eating

You'll often hear people in the keto community talking about macros. *Macro* is short for *macronutrient,* and macronutrients are the nutrients your body needs to thrive. The three main macronutrients are fat, protein, and carbohydrates.

Macros are usually expressed as percentages. Common macros for a standard American diet are about 35 percent fat, 15 percent protein, and 50 percent carbohydrates. Macros for a ketogenic diet are usually about 75 percent fat, 20 percent protein, and 5 percent carbohydrates.

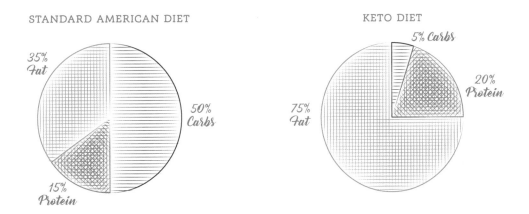

STANDARD AMERICAN DIET

35% Fat
50% Carbs
15% Protein

KETO DIET

5% Carbs
20% Protein
75% Fat

You can use an online keto calculator to calculate your personal macros, and you can use apps such as MyFitnessPal, Keto Diet App, and Carb Manager to track your daily percentages. Some people find that this approach works well in the beginning to help them grasp the keto lifestyle, and then they transition to intuitive keto.

It is often referred to as "lazy keto," but I prefer the term *intuitive.* This is my preferred approach. I have tried both, and intuitive keto is what I decided I could maintain long term. People who intuitively eat keto track net carbs, usually 20 to 50 grams per day, but keep a mental count instead of writing it down or using an app. For me, it's about listening to my body and learning what makes me feel good. It requires patience and a willingness to make changes as necessary. I eat normal-sized portions of allowable foods (see pages 24 and 25). I make conscious decisions about what to eat, and I eat until satisfied but not overly stuffed. Also, I no longer mindlessly snack.

I've found that the method you prefer can greatly depend on your personality type. Some people truly enjoy tracking macros! You have to know yourself and your triggers. Set yourself up for success. For me, counting every day felt too restrictive and led to bingeing. Intuitive keto is more sustainable for me. I know others who succeed on keto only when they count macros. Sometimes it takes trying both ways to decide. I've said it before and I'll say it again: keto is not one-size-fits-all. We are individuals, and we have individual needs. Use the method that works better for you!

Here are some tips to help with the transition:

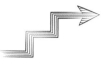

KEEP IT SIMPLE.

Overcomplicating things can lead to frustration and cause you to throw in the towel before you even get started.

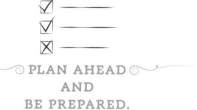

PLAN AHEAD
AND
BE PREPARED.

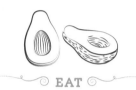

EAT
REAL FOOD

and avoid processed and prepackaged foods.

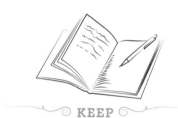

KEEP
A DAILY JOURNAL

and write down how you're feeling, what was hard for you, and what was good.

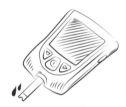

Testing for ketosis

Are you in ketosis? These are the most common ways to tell:

- **How you feel**—This is my preferred method. When I am in ketosis, I have increased energy and better metal clarity, and my hunger and sugar cravings diminish. It's an overall good feeling, and once you've experienced it, you'll know it! One downside is that you may experience bad breath, sometimes known as keto breath.

- **Ketone urine strips**—Ketostix, sold at most drugstores, are strips that change color if ketones are present in your urine. They aren't always accurate because ketone levels in the urine don't necessarily match ketone levels in the blood.

- **Blood ketone meter**—The most expensive but the most accurate way to measure ketosis is to analyze your blood for ketones. You use a lancet to prick your finger and then test your blood with a meter. Optimal readings are between 0.5 and 3.0 mmol/L.

You certainly don't have to use either of these testing methods. Many people have success by eating a ketogenic diet alone and do not track ketones.

Tracking your progress

Weight loss is a common goal for people following a ketogenic diet, but there are other measures of success as well. Here are some tips for tracking your progress:

- **Weigh yourself no more than once a week;** daily water weight fluctuations can be discouraging. I'm not saying that losing weight isn't important, but don't let it be your only measure of success.

- **Take your measurements.** Sometimes you'll discover inches lost even when the number on the scale hasn't moved.

- **Take a lot of pictures of yourself before starting keto and throughout your journey.** Photos showing your progress can be very motivating!

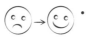

- **Take stock of how you feel.** Are you feeling better overall? Do you have more mental clarity?

Non-scale victories, also known as NSVs, are my favorite! It's not all about the number on the scale; pay attention to your non-scale victories, too. It's the little changes you notice along the way that will help you stay motivated and change your quality of life for the better. Here are a few examples:

- Clothing getting looser
- Clothing sizes going down
- Someone noticing that you've lost weight
- Airplane seatbelt fitting without an extender

- Having more energy
- Feeling healthier and stronger
- Being able to do more physical activity without feeling overexerted
- Anything else that improves your quality of life!

Dealing with slow or no weight loss

I get so many questions from people who are discouraged about not losing weight or not losing it fast enough. This isn't a race. Yes, you want to make sure you are progressing, but everyone is different and loses weight at different rates. Sometimes I think people get discouraged because they see testimonies of people losing 100 pounds in six months on keto. While I've seen that happen, I see a lot more people like myself who lose weight slower. Progress is progress, no matter how long it takes. I used to get frustrated, but eventually I realized that as long as I didn't quit, I found success.

Finding encouragement to stay the course

My hope in sharing these words is that someone reading this will be encouraged. If you feel moved by anything I've said, then this section is for you. You are worth it—you matter!

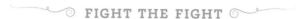

FIGHT THE FIGHT

The fight is worth it. You're worth it. If you fall down, get back up and try again. I know it sounds cliché, but staying in the fight truly has been the secret to my success. People always want to know the secret. It's not a huge deal; it's about consistently making the right choices. The little things add up. As with any lifestyle change, consistency is key. I wrote this book for people who follow a ketogenic lifestyle, but the same rules for success apply no matter which method you choose. It's about deciding you want it and how badly you want it.

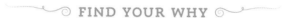

FIND YOUR WHY

Discover your why. Why do you want to do this? Your why has to be so big that quitting is not an option. Not everyone's why will be weight loss. Some people try keto for health reasons. Some are looking for a better quality of life. There will be roadblocks along the way. You may have to tweak some things to find out what truly works for you. Patience is required! Dig your heels in deep and determine in your heart that you will not make excuses or give up. Your why needs to drive you. If you don't really know your why or don't have a strong why, spend some time defining it. Journal every day. Read over your journal entries, and the things that are important to you will begin to stand out.

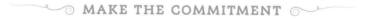

MAKE THE COMMITMENT

I use the word *commit* a lot. Commitment is staying loyal to what you said you would do after the mood in which you said it has passed. Deciding to commit is the most important thing you will ever do. No matter the path you choose, you have to commit, because there will be days when you won't want to do it. There will be days when you couldn't care less. Those are the days when your commitment has to override your feelings. Feelings are subject to change every day, sometimes multiple times a day! Staying committed is the most important thing you'll ever do for yourself. Small changes add up to big results over time.

REDEFINE SUCCESS

How do you define success? Success means something different for everyone. In a world where skinniness is idealized, skinny used to be the measure of success for me. I have never been skinny, nor will I ever be skinny. And you know what? That's okay. And if you are skinny, that is okay, too! You see, my measure of success has evolved over the years, thankfully. As an overweight kid, all I ever wanted was to fit in. When I had my first real success with weight loss, I thought success was about losing the weight. After losing and regaining weight so many times over the years, I realized that weight loss could not be the only way I measure success. When I lost weight, I still felt incomplete; I was never satisfied. I enjoyed the newfound attention, but I was counting on the weight loss to change me, to make me happy. It never made me happy or made me feel any more worthy. I'm sure age has a way of changing these feelings, but now I measure my success not by my weight, but by the quality of my life. Getting to this place has been so freeing!

FIND BALANCE

Throughout my life, I've been sick and I've been healthy. I've been morbidly obese and I've been at an average weight. But what I feel now is balance. That's what was missing! I feel more at peace with where I am physically and emotionally than I ever have before. Even though I have a lot of physical flaws and some loose skin, I am content. I am not perfect; I still have days when I look in the mirror and nothing satisfies me, and I can't find anything to wear that I think looks good. Some days I feel a lot bigger than I really am. It's a mental thing. I am a normal person and I still have struggles, but they do not define me. A clothing size does not define me. A number on a scale does not define me. I am so much more than that. You are so much more than that.

You will have a different why and a different goal than I do, but my hope is that you will be intentional and stay on the path to what you define as success, no matter how long it takes! Be willing to try and try again. Be willing to make the necessary tweaks to find the approach that works for your body. We are all unique individuals, and the same path will not work for everyone, but there is a path for you. Because of my struggles and successes, I now believe with my whole heart that if I can do it, anyone can! Your only limit is you.

I know you may be thinking to yourself, *Well, yes, this all sounds good, but how do you get to that place?* I've had many people ask me that very question. I wish I had a magic answer. You have to find your motivation. For me, I got to a point of desperation. I was so exhausted and desperate for change—for lasting change! I was so tired of being sick and tired and of being on the roller coaster of food addiction. Like I said, I'm not perfect, but the difference now is that I have developed some coping mechanisms. I used to think that if I had a bad day, it was over. Now, if I have a bad day, I let it be just that—a bad day. I don't let it carry over into several consecutive bad days, weeks, or even months.

SEEK SUPPORT—
AND BE SUPPORTIVE OF OTHERS

Developing a strong support system is very important. I am thankful for my husband, family, and friends who have supported me unconditionally through my highs and lows. I know that not everyone gets this kind of support at home. Sometimes you have to look elsewhere for it. Online keto communities such as those found on Instagram, Facebook, and Reddit became a huge source of inspiration for me and many others. I am thankful for the connections I have made with people who get it—people who have been through the same kinds of struggles and are still going through them.

When it comes to the people you live with, sometimes you have to lead by example. You can't change them overnight if they aren't interested in change. At first, my husband wasn't interested in changing how he ate. He supported me in the ways that he could, but he didn't want to make changes for himself. When I finally decided to fully commit, things changed for me, not just physically but also mentally. I became stronger and more focused. I think my family and friends could see that. People in my life started making changes, too—not because I asked them to, but because they could see the differences in me and wanted to experience that kind of change for themselves. My husband started his keto journey in June 2015. It wasn't always easy for him. There were a lot of moments when he almost quit, but he hung in there and has found success in both losing weight and improving his health markers!

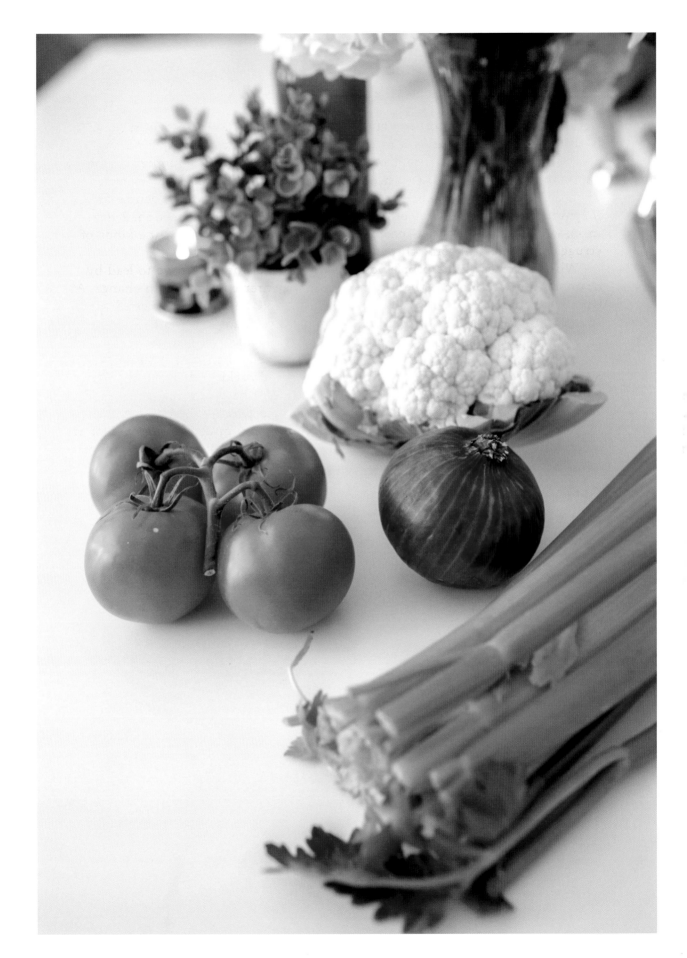

Eating and Cooking Keto

On the opposite page is a basic grocery list of the foods that I often buy. It serves to show you just how many food choices you have on keto. It doesn't have to be complicated! I live in a rural area, and most of these items are easy for me to find.

Keto allowable foods

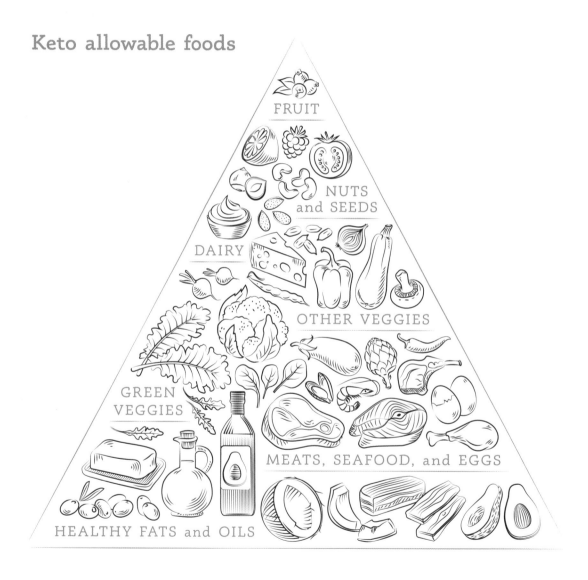

FRUIT

NUTS and SEEDS

DAIRY

OTHER VEGGIES

GREEN VEGGIES

MEATS, SEAFOOD, and EGGS

HEALTHY FATS and OILS

MEATS & EGGS

Beef *(all cuts)*

Lamb

Pork *(chops, roast, and tenderloin)*

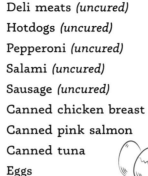

Venison

Chicken *(all cuts)*

Turkey

Fish and shellfish

Bacon

Deli meats *(uncured)*

Hotdogs *(uncured)*

Pepperoni *(uncured)*

Salami *(uncured)*

Sausage *(uncured)*

Canned chicken breast

Canned pink salmon

Canned tuna

Eggs

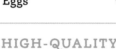

VEGGIES
(fresh & frozen)

Artichokes

Asparagus

Baby spinach

Bell peppers

Braising greens, such as collards, kale, and Swiss chard

Broccoli

Brussels sprouts

Cabbage

Cauliflower

Celery

Cucumbers

Eggplant

Garlic

Green beans

Green onions *(aka scallions)*

Hot peppers

Jalapeños

Lettuce

Mushrooms

Onions *(red, white, and yellow)*

Radishes

Rhubarb

Salad greens

Spaghetti squash

Yellow squash

Zucchini

HIGH-QUALITY FATS & OILS

(see pages 27 and 28)

FRUITS & BERRIES

Avocados

Blackberries

Blueberries

Lemons

Limes

Raspberries

Strawberries

Tomatoes

NUTS, SEEDS, & NUT BUTTERS

Almonds

Cashews

Hazelnuts

Macadamia nuts

Peanuts

Pecans

Pistachios

Shelled sunflower seeds

Walnuts

Natural almond butter *(unsalted and unsweetened)*

Natural peanut butter *(unsalted and unsweetened)*

DAIRY

Butter

Cheese *(full fat)*

Cream cheese

Heavy cream

Sour cream

MISCELLANEOUS

Broth

Dill relish *(no sugar added)*

Ketchup *(no sugar added)*

Mayonnaise

Nondairy milks *(see page 27)*

Salad dressings *(full-fat, low-carb, and without added sugars)*

Olives

Parmesan cheese crisps *(see "A few of my favorite products," page 285)*

Pickles *(no sugar added)*

Pork rinds

Ketogenic flours *(see page 26)*

Unsweetened coconut flakes and shredded coconut

KETOGENIC SEASONINGS & FLAVORINGS

Herbs, fresh and dried

Ketogenic sweeteners *(see page 29)*

Natural flavor extracts *(see page 27)*

Salt, all flavors and textures *(pink Himalayan salt is the type I use most)*

Spices

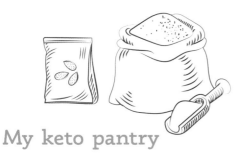

My keto pantry

Let's face it: on a keto lifestyle, you need certain pantry items in order to make foods that keep you from getting bored and help you stay on track. These are the necessities that I always keep on hand for keto cooking and baking. If they are hard to find in your area, don't worry, because most of these items can be ordered online. Amazon and Netrition have competitive prices. I usually check several sites to make sure I'm getting the best deal. Many of these foods are shelf-stable items. Some are frozen or refrigerated.

Almond flour—Finely ground blanched almond flour is my favorite and most-used flour for low-carb baking. I often purchase it in bulk.

Coconut flour—Coconut flour doesn't work the same way as almond flour; it is very absorbent and needs more liquid. It is a little tricky to get used to but is great for low-carb baking. It's frequently used by people who have nut allergies. It absorbs moisture, so it's best stored in an airtight container. I store mine at room temperature.

Chia seeds—Chia is a superfood that is packed with antioxidants, fiber, and fat. The seeds can be used in foods and drinks. My personal favorite use for chia seeds is pudding! See my recipe on page 244.

Golden flaxseed meal—Flaxseed meal adds texture to ketogenic baked goods such as Skillet Cornbread (page 74). I prefer the golden variety because it is more visually appealing and tastes better. It's also rich in omega-3 fatty acids and fiber.

Oat fiber—Not to be confused with oat flour, oat fiber has zero carbs and adds a nice texture and flavor to certain low-carb baked goods, such as zucchini bread (find my recipe on page 82). I use Trim Healthy Momma brand.

Psyllium husks—These are used in low-carb and gluten-free baking to add a breadlike texture. I use Indus Organics brand.

Xanthan gum—Not absolutely necessary but great to have. You can use it to thicken sauces and soups or as a binder to give low-carb baked goods elasticity and volume so that they more closely resemble conventional baked goods. Sometimes I even use it in blended protein shakes and milkshakes to thicken them and improve the texture. It takes only a tiny amount, so use it sparingly.

Flavor extracts—Extracts can give foods and drinks the flavors of higher-carb foods without the added carbs. You need only a very small amount. Some of my favorite flavors are vanilla, sweet corn, maple, orange, and coconut. Of course, my most-used extract is vanilla. Search for extracts that are pure and naturally flavored, without added sugars.

Nondairy milks—There are many uses for unsweetened nondairy milks such as almond milk and full-fat coconut milk on a keto diet. They are often used as a replacement for dairy milk in recipes or as a creamer for coffee.

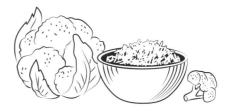

Frozen riced cauliflower—You will need a convenient keto replacement for high-carb sides. This is my go-to choice for ease of use. See "Low-carb swaps" on page 38 for more ideas.

Unflavored collagen peptides—Collagen is good blended into coffee and smoothies. There are health benefits to using a good grass-fed collagen, including improvements in skin, hair, nails, and joints.

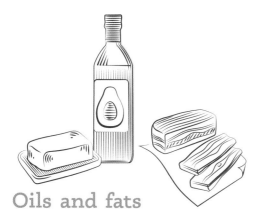

Oils and fats

Keto is a high-fat way of eating, so it's important to use good-quality fats and oils.

Bacon drippings (aka bacon fat or grease) are wonderful for frying and add a unique depth of flavor to whatever you are cooking. It even makes a great salad dressing! Anytime you make bacon, drain the grease and save it. You can keep it on the counter like my grandma did, but it goes rancid much faster than if it is stored in an airtight container in the refrigerator, where it will keep for up to six months.

Butter has so many uses in a ketogenic lifestyle—everything from coffee to frying eggs. Not all butters are created equal, although I used to think so. Grass-fed butter is best. Kerrygold brand grass-fed butter is my favorite for its quality and flavor. Note that I use salted butter in the recipes in this book. If you prefer to use unsalted butter, you may need to increase the amount of salt called for in the recipes just slightly.

Ghee, a kind of clarified butter, can be a good option for those who are sensitive to dairy and lactose. It has a high smoke point, making it a good choice for frying.

Lard has a neutral flavor and a high smoke point, which makes it good for frying. Look for non-hydrogenated lard. It is a traditional Southern cooking and baking fat, used for everything from fried chicken to biscuits.

Avocado oil has a mild flavor with a high smoke point of up to 450°F. I frequently use it for deep-frying.

Coconut oil has a high smoke point that makes it good for frying, but its coconut flavor makes it less favorable for some recipes.

Extra-virgin olive oil is useful for roasting vegetables and for salad dressings. It is not a great choice for frying because of its lower smoke point.

MCT oil is a good way to add healthy fat to your ketogenic diet. Medium-chain triglycerides (MCTs) are naturally occurring fatty acids in coconut oil. MCT oil is flavorless and can be added to coffee, smoothies, and salad dressings.

DEEP-FRYING TIPS

For frying, you can use a deep-fryer or a large, deep, heavy pot. I use a 6-quart Dutch oven. It helps maintain the temperature of the oil and cooks foods evenly, and the depth of the pot helps keep messes to a minimum.

When choosing oils for deep-frying, it is essential to use an oil with a high smoke point. Above you can read more about different oils.

It's important to maintain a consistent temperature when deep-frying. If the temperature of the oil is too low, the food will absorb the oil and become soggy instead of crispy. I use a candy thermometer to monitor and maintain a consistent temperature. Adding too much food to the oil at one time will lower the temperature quickly; that is why many recipes call for deep-frying foods in batches so as not to overcrowd the pot. When frying food in batches, make sure that the oil has returned to the ideal temperature before adding the next batch of food.

Foods should be completely submerged in oil when frying. That is why I give the quantity of oil to be used in inches rather than listing a volume amount in the ingredient list. This ensures the correct depth of oil for the food being fried, regardless of the diameter of the pot used.

It's important not to overfill the pot with oil so as to avoid a grease fire; a good general rule is never to fill a pot more than halfway full. Watch the oil throughout the entire cooking process; never walk away from hot oil.

You could use a fresh batch of oil every time, but keto-friendly oils are expensive. Oil used for frying can be reused as long as it's stored properly. Allow the oil to cool completely. Use a fine-mesh strainer to strain the oil into a container with a lid; a glass jar works well. Store the oil in a cool, dry place. (It does not have to be refrigerated.) If the oil looks cloudy or has a bad smell, it's time to discard it.

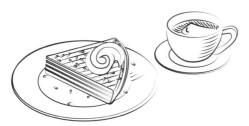

Sweeteners

Not all sugar-free sweeteners are created equal. It's important to look for natural sweeteners with a low glycemic index (GI), meaning that they do not raise blood sugar. Stay away from artificial sweeteners, which may actually increase blood glucose levels and can cause stomach irritability in some people. Avoid sweetener packets, as most contain carbs and dextrose.

BETTER SWEETENERS WITH A LOW GI

These are the keto-friendly sweeteners that I recommend:

- **Erythritol and erythritol blends**—granular and confectioners'-style. You can grind granular erythritol to make powdered.

- **Monk fruit and monk fruit blended with erythritol**

- **Stevia**—liquid and powdered

- **Xylitol**—A fine low-GI choice for a ketogenic lifestyle, but I avoid it because it can be hazardous to pets if ingested.

LESS-DESIRABLE SWEETENERS

These artificial sweeteners are known to have unpleasant or dangerous side effects and raise blood sugar in some people. Maltitol, for instance, has been found to cause headaches and stomach irritability.

- **Aspartame**

- **Maltitol**

- **Saccharin**

- **Sucralose**

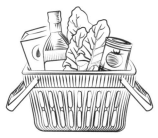

Where I shop and what I buy

I live in a small town, so I understand the challenges that some people face in finding popular keto foods locally. I shop at my local grocery stores weekly. Then, at least once a month, I make a trip to a larger town over an hour away to shop at stores like Aldi, Costco, and Trader Joe's. I load my car with coolers filled with ice. Stocking up on my favorite and most-used products is worth the extra effort.

ALDI

Bacon

Butter

Eggs

Heavy cream

Nuts and seeds

Oils

Organic apple cider vinegar

Organic produce—selection varies seasonally

Pepperoni

Pork rinds

Prosciutto

Salami

Sausage

Sour cream

Specialty cheeses—hard and sliced

Uncured nitrate-free lunch meats

COSTCO

Almond flour

Avocado oil

Avocados

Bacon

Berries

Bulk spices

Canned chicken breast

Canned sardines

Canned tuna

Cheeses—hard and sliced

Chicken breasts

Chicken wings

Coconut oil

Coffee

Eggs

English cucumbers

Extra-virgin olive oil

Frozen broccoli florets

Frozen riced cauliflower

Green nonstarchy vegetables

Ground beef

Guacamole in single-serving cups

Hamburgers

Hard-boiled eggs

Heavy cream

Kerrygold butter

Lunch meats

Marinara sauce

Mayonnaise

Nuts—almonds, macadamia nuts, pecans, walnuts

Organic salsa

Pimento cheese

Pork chops

Pork tenderloin

Queso fresco

Raw almond butter

Ribs

Rotisserie chicken

Steaks

String cheese

Tomatoes

Uncured hotdogs

Whisps cheese crisps

Wild Alaskan salmon

TRADER JOE'S

Trader Joe's sells a store brand of most of the items below. Anytime there's a choice, I choose the store brand because I've consistently found it to be of high quality.

Almond flour

Aluminum-free baking powder

Avocado oil

Avocados

Bacon ends and pieces

Beef sticks

Bell peppers

Berries

Canned wild salmon

Cheeses—hard and sliced

Chia seeds

Coconut aminos

Coconut flour

Coconut milk (full-fat)

Coconut oil

Coconut oil spray

Dips and spreads

Extra-virgin olive oil

Flaxseed meal

Fresh riced broccoli

Frozen shaved Brussels sprouts

Green nonstarchy vegetables

Heavy cream

Kerrygold butter

Liquid stevia

Mascarpone cheese

Mini sweet peppers

Montezuma unsweetened chocolate bars (100% cacao)

Nuts

Olives

Organic broth

Organic peanut butter

Oven-baked cheese bites

Persian cucumbers

Pork belly

Psyllium husks

Raw almond butter

Riced cauliflower, frozen and fresh

Sesame oil

Spaghetti squash

Sparkling water

Spices—21 seasoning salute, everyday seasoning, everything bagel seasoning, garlic salt grinder, onion salt, pink Himalayan salt, seasoning salt

Tomatoes

Unsweetened cocoa powder

Unsweetened coconut flakes

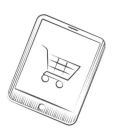

ONLINE

There are also some things that I order online. I always cross-check prices and usually find the best deals on Amazon and Netrition. When I can't get to the stores listed above, I buy shelf-stable pantry items online.

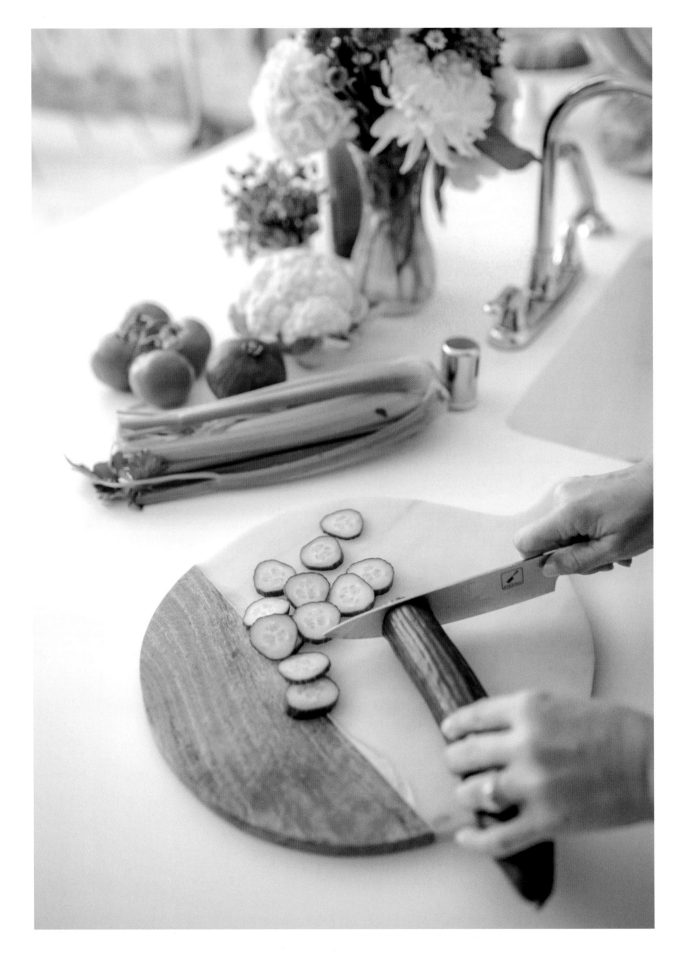

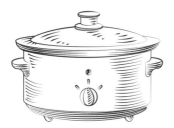

My favorite kitchen tools

I love kitchen gadgets and small appliances. This section lists my favorite and most-used items. This list assumes that your kitchen is already equipped with the basics: a set of pots and pans, some baking dishes, mixing bowls, wooden spoons, cutting boards, and so on. Some of the tools listed here are necessary (or extremely helpful) for making many of the recipes in this book, and others are just nice to have.

Cast-iron skillet—There's nothing like a well-seasoned cast-iron skillet. Seasoned cast iron has a coating of oil that protects it from rust and creates a nonstick cooking surface. These pans are durable; if you take good care of them, they can last a lifetime and be passed down for generations to come. They hold up to high heat and distribute heat evenly, which makes them ideal for searing meats, frying, and roasting. I like how cast iron easily goes from stovetop to oven. I most frequently use my 12-inch and 10-inch cast-iron skillets. Never put them in the dishwasher. Hand wash with hot water and a stiff bristle brush and a pan scraper if needed. Towel dry immediately and then apply a light layer of your preferred cooking oil. Store in a dry place.

Enameled Dutch oven, 6-quart—Another kitchen investment that's made to last. An enameled Dutch oven is perfect for soups and stews, as well as for deep-frying, simmering, and braising. It keeps food at a consistent temperature for even cooking and is easy to clean. Depending on the brand you choose, these pots can be quite expensive, but Lodge makes a budget-priced Dutch oven that's nice quality.

Slow cooker—A lot of people love their slow cookers because of their ease of use. Another thing I like about the slow cooker is how it brings out the flavor in foods and helps tenderize less-expensive cuts of meat.

Waffle maker—You can use this handy little appliance to make the low-carb waffles on page 64. You don't need to buy an expensive one; I paid around $20 for my waffle maker. Remember to spray it with oil before each use to ensure that the waffles don't stick.

Blender, immersion and countertop—My immersion blender (aka stick blender) is one of my most beloved kitchen tools. I use it for just about everything that needs blending. My favorite use is for milkshakes and smoothies. With an immersion blender, it's easy to blend your drink right in the cup. I also use my immersion blender to blend soups right in the pot. Not having to transfer hot soup to a countertop blender saves you a lot of time and hassle. The best part of an immersion blender is the easy cleanup. The end pops off and can be put in the dishwasher. There's hardly a need for a full-size countertop blender, although I like those, too, for larger jobs such as making smoothies and shakes for more than one person.

Food processor—Not a must-have appliance, but a food processor is versatile and sure does make some kitchen prep tasks easier! A food processor is great if you do a lot of chopping, shredding, and slicing. A great use is making your own nut butters. You can also use it for purees and sauces.

Hand mixer—An electric hand mixer is inexpensive and easy to clean. You can put the attachments in the dishwasher. I use my hand mixer for smaller jobs that don't require a stand mixer.

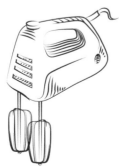

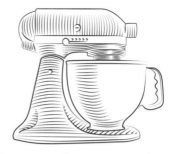

Stand mixer—This was my first costly small kitchen appliance purchase. I considered it an investment, and it has paid off; my KitchenAid stand mixer has lasted over twelve years so far. It's not a necessary item, but it's so nice to have for larger jobs and when you want to mix ingredients hands-free. The possibilities for its uses are endless, and there are so many attachments you can add. I like to use my stand mixer with the dough hook attachment to quickly combine the ingredients for meatloaf and sausage. Any recipe in this book that calls for a hand mixer can be made using a stand mixer instead.

Baking sheets (aka cookie sheets)—I use these to bake drop biscuits and shortcakes. My baking sheets are 21 by 15 inches.

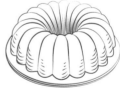

Bundt pan, 12-cup—I love Bundt pans and own three of them. Of course, Bundt pans are great for cakes, but they have other uses, too. I use mine for meatloaf and pull-apart keto breads and as a mold to make an ice ring for punch.

Loaf pan, 9 by 5-inch—A loaf pan can be used for breads as well as for savory recipes such as meatloaf.

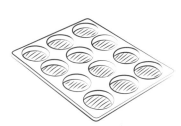

Muffin pan, 12-cup—Standard-size muffin pans are great to have for making muffins, of course, as well as my Bacon Cheeseburger Mini Meatloaves (see page 166). For many recipes, individual silicone muffin cups can be used in place of a muffin pan, if desired.

Parchment paper—I use parchment paper in many of my recipes. Parchment paper tops the list of my favorite kitchen items because it makes cleanup so easy; nothing sticks to it! I love to cook but dislike scrubbing pans. Don't confuse it with wax paper. If you don't have parchment paper, no worries—in most cases you can grease the pan or use foil or a silicone baking mat instead.

Sheet pans (aka rimmed baking sheets)—I use these almost every day for sheet pan dinners, roasted vegetables, pizza, and so much more. They're inexpensive, too; I've even purchased old high-quality sheet pans at thrift stores. I use a standard-size sheet pan, 18 by 13 inches.

Springform pan, 9-inch and/or 10-inch—This type of bakeware features sides that can be removed from the base. The most common use is for cheesecake.

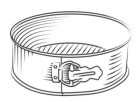

Silicone baking cups, silicone candy mold, silicone mat—Silicone is nice to own because nothing sticks to it, and unlike parchment paper, it is reusable, making it more cost-effective over time. A silicone candy mold comes in handy when making the Dark Chocolate Coconut Fat Bombs on page 246, though 1-inch foil candy liners can also be used.

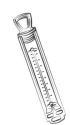

Candy thermometer—I use this inexpensive tool for deep-frying and for the Southern Boiled Custard recipe on page 264.

Kitchen shears—I love a good pair of kitchen shears. They're great for opening food packages and snipping herbs. You can even use them to cut up bacon. Raw bacon is greasy and can be a bit slippery to work with when chopping it for a recipe. Kitchen shears make the task much easier.

Knives—You don't have to spend hundreds of dollars on kitchen knives. Some people might argue that point, but I've never owned expensive knives, and I have managed quite well. I don't buy the cheapest knives; I buy a few moderately priced knives and take good care of them. Just keep them sharpened and do not put them in the dishwasher, which will dull them.

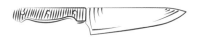

Mesh skimmer—This inexpensive little tool makes it easier and safer to remove foods from hot oil when deep-frying.

NICE-TO-HAVE GADGETS

Food scale—This is another item that you don't absolutely have to have, but a scale comes in handy when you need an exact weight for accuracy. Scales are especially useful for people who like to track their foods closely. A scale doesn't take up much space and can be inexpensive. There are some nice food scales online for as little as $10.

Frother—I love having a handheld battery-operated frother to mix cream into coffee. You can also use it to blend powders and oils into any drink. It's not strong enough to thoroughly whip a bulletproof coffee, but it's perfect for small jobs. I've seen frothers for as little as $3.

Instant Pot—The Instant Pot is fairly new on the scene, but the pressure cooker concept isn't new. This isn't your grandma's pressure cooker, however. I love how fast and easy it is to use. Don't be intimidated by the Instant Pot—it's completely safe to use. My favorite thing to cook in my Instant Pot is hard-boiled eggs. They are effortless, and the shells slide right off! The Instant Pot also has a slow cooker function if you don't have the budget or the storage space for two separate appliances.

Spiral slicer—This tool makes zucchini and other vegetable noodles. These slicers can be purchased at most stores and in a wide range of prices. I bought mine at a discount store for less than $10, and it works wonderfully.

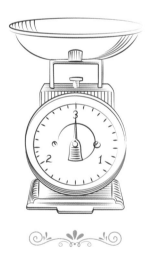

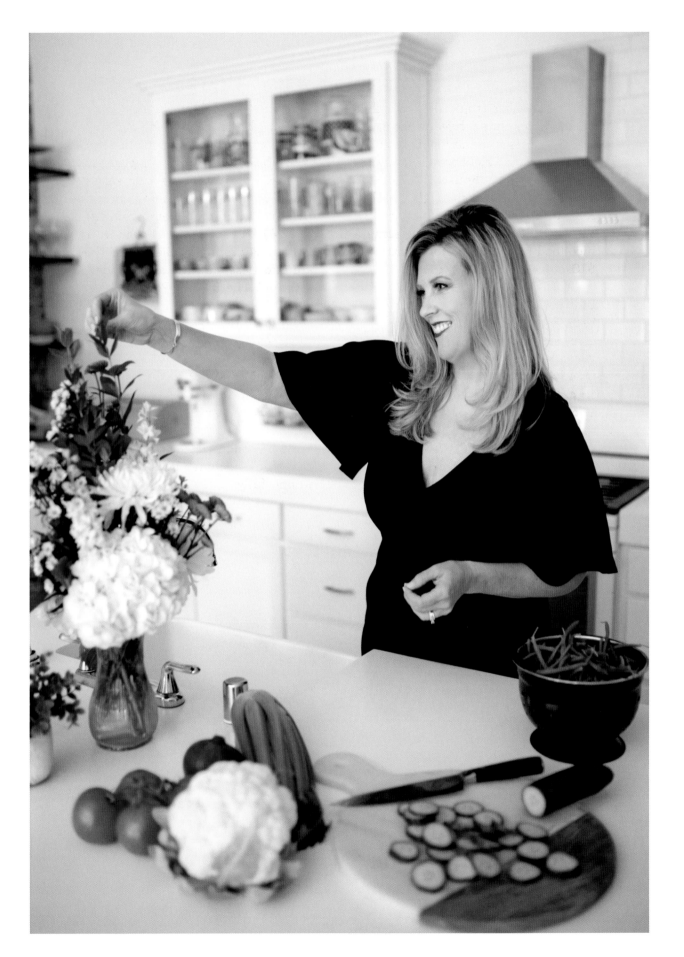

Practical Keto Tips

Low-carb swaps

There are many delicious low-carb food swaps that will make it easier for you to stick to your ketogenic lifestyle. Here are the swaps that I've found to be the most useful:

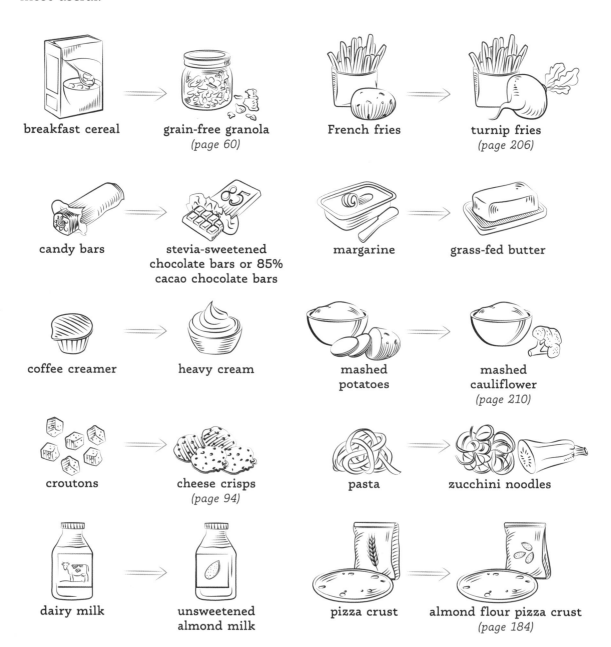

breakfast cereal → grain-free granola *(page 60)*

French fries → turnip fries *(page 206)*

candy bars → stevia-sweetened chocolate bars or 85% cacao chocolate bars

margarine → grass-fed butter

coffee creamer → heavy cream

mashed potatoes → mashed cauliflower *(page 210)*

croutons → cheese crisps *(page 94)*

pasta → zucchini noodles

dairy milk → unsweetened almond milk

pizza crust → almond flour pizza crust *(page 184)*

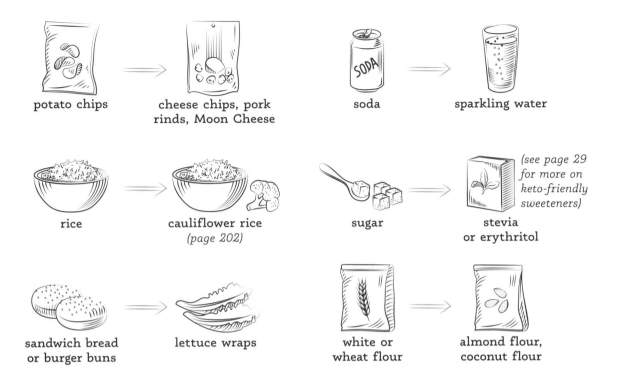

potato chips → cheese chips, pork rinds, Moon Cheese

soda → sparkling water

rice → cauliflower rice
(page 202)

sugar → stevia or erythritol

(see page 29 for more on keto-friendly sweeteners)

sandwich bread or burger buns → lettuce wraps

white or wheat flour → almond flour, coconut flour

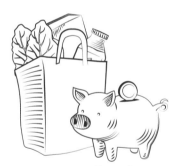

Keto on a budget

Keto is expensive, right? It doesn't have to be. You can absolutely follow a ketogenic lifestyle on a budget; you just need a plan!

When I first started eating keto, I paid no mind to the quality of the food I was eating. I just wanted to make sure it was low-carb and that I got results. Over time, I've learned a lot, and now I make better food choices whenever I can. I've found that when I eat more high-quality whole foods, I feel better.

As far as costs go, do the best you can wherever you can. I would hate for someone not to make any changes just because of the cost. If you can't afford grass-fed meats and organic vegetables, make the best choices that work for your budget! Eat as healthily as you can and don't let price be an excuse to choose unhealthy food. Think about the health issues that often stem from eating poorly. Those will cost you money in the long run. Eating well is a long-term investment in your health!

Here are some useful tips for your food budget:

- **Clip coupons and research sale circulars each week.**

- **Make a list before you go shopping, and stick to your list.** I am guilty of not doing this from time to time, but when I do, I spend a lot less money. Following a list also helps prevent waste because you buy only what you need.

- **Stock up!** When your favorite meats are on sale, buy extras and freeze them. We have a chest freezer in the garage for storing meats. The same goes for other foods that can be stored for a longer time: find them at low prices and stock up.

- **Buy frozen vegetables.** Some vegetables are best eaten fresh, but many are wonderful purchased frozen. I frequently buy frozen broccoli and cauliflower, for example.

- **Buy in bulk if you can get a membership to a wholesale club such as Costco or Sam's Club.** If you shop there often like I do, the membership pays for itself. I make a trip to Costco at least once a month. There, I get the best deals on bulk almond flour, avocado oil, and nuts. You can find my full Costco shopping list on page 30.

- **Shop online.** I find great deals online, and I cross-check prices on several websites before purchasing an item. Amazon and Netrition are two of my go-to sources.

- **Join a local food co-op** to save money on freshly grown produce and buy food from bulk bins, allowing you to purchase just the amount you need.

- **Plant your own garden.** If space is a factor, consider a small container garden on your patio.

- **Plan meals and batch cook.** I like to double or triple recipes to have leftovers for the week. Some meals are good for freezing, too. See page 51 for ideas.

- **Find other ways to cut back to allow room in your budget for better-quality meats and vegetables.** An example would be buying less coffee from a coffee shop and making your own coffee drinks instead. Another would be eating out less often on workdays and packing your lunch instead.

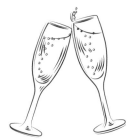

Special-occasion keto

Celebrations and special occasions are the reason some people (myself included) have been known to, as they say, fall off the wagon. Some call it a "cheat meal," but I don't like that phrase because it implies that you're doing something wrong. I prefer to call it "going off plan for a meal" or something like that. Whether or not to go off plan is a personal decision, so I'll leave that to you, with no judgment. For me, it can be a slippery slope, and I've learned that the hard way. You have to know yourself, your history, and your patterns. I believe there's a difference between thoughtfully deciding to have an off-plan meal and indulging in a spur-of-the-moment "cheat." It's the difference between being in control and being out of control.

Using every holiday and gathering you are invited to as an excuse to go off plan makes it impossible to be consistent. There's always something to celebrate! Over time, I've learned that for me, it's easier to stay on plan. There are ways to do that and not feel deprived. There's not a lot you can do about a function where you have no control over the food, but you can control how you react. Focus on the atmosphere and the people you care about and be in the moment!

Here are some other tips for special occasions:

- **Plan ahead.** There's nothing worse than feeling deprived; this is what you want to avoid.

- **Offer to host the gathering.** Serving as host gives you control over the food. And many of the recipes in this book would please anyone, no matter what their eating style!

- **Eat a healthy snack before you go.** Don't go to an event starving.

- **Stay hydrated** by drinking plenty of water.

- **Ask if you can bring a dish that you can eat.** If you can't, you may be able to pack a snack in your bag. I've done this lots of times!

- **Decide what you are going to do before you get there.** Going off plan is an individual choice; do what you know will make you feel good in the long run. Set limits for yourself so that you do not overindulge. If you don't think you have the self-control to do so, then it is probably wiser not to go off plan.

- **Get right back to your routine as soon as possible.** If you do go off keto, whether you intended to or not, don't dwell on it or beat yourself up! Keep moving forward.

A WORD ABOUT DESSERT

There are a lot of wonderful keto desserts in this book, but if you are new to keto, it can be helpful to cut out treats temporarily—yes, even keto desserts. In my experience, the longer you go without triggering your brain to anticipate sweets, the more likely your cravings for sweets will diminish. Then you can start incorporating a few on-plan treats. This approach is especially helpful if you find that you are addicted to sugar. You'll be surprised at how little it takes to satisfy you after cutting out sugar for a few weeks. I've done this myself, and it has helped me tremendously. Now I can eat a small portion of dessert and feel satisfied—I no longer feel out of control when it comes to sweets. Of course, this is just a suggestion. Make an informed decision about dessert based on knowing yourself and your tendencies.

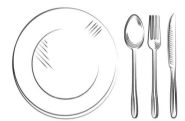

Keeping it keto at restaurants

We used to eat out a lot. We ate huge meals, always ordering an appetizer, salad, main dish, and sometimes dessert, even if we were too full! We still enjoy dining out, but these days I prefer making my own food at home. That way, I have more control over what goes into it. I can make a wide variety of keto-friendly dishes that we can't get at a restaurant, and the homemade versions are more satisfying.

That being said, I understand that sometimes you need to eat out. I do enjoy the social aspect of dining with friends and family, and I try to make my visits to restaurants more about that. And it is possible to enjoy a great meal out, stay on plan, and not feel deprived.

I used to be terrified of eating out while trying to stay keto. It can be tricky, but the good news is that the more you do it, the easier it gets. You'll find yourself looking at menus in a whole new way. Now I focus on what I *can* have instead of what I can't have. You can take me to just about any restaurant, and I'll find something I can eat and enjoy! Here are my tips for eating out on keto:

- **Planning ahead is key!** If possible, look at the restaurant menu before you go and decide what you'll order in advance.

- **Don't be shy about making special requests and substitutions.** Just ask nicely, and you'll be surprised at how far a lot of places will go to accommodate your needs.

- **Stick to foods that aren't breaded,** and pick nonstarchy vegetables for sides.

- **Use dressing sparingly or ask for it on the side.** Order full-fat dressings. Some salad dressings and other condiments have added sugars. I stick to ranch, Caesar, or blue cheese dressing. You could also ask for oil and vinegar for your salad.

- Ketchup contains added sugars and carbs. Use mustard or mayo instead. I've also been known to bring my own no-sugar-added ketchup to restaurants!

- Use caution when ordering dishes that have sauces. Ask if the sauce has sugar or flour in it before ordering.

- Ask questions before ordering soup. A lot of soups use flour as a thickener, and some contain sugar.

- If possible, ask the server to not bring the bread or chips.

- Breakfast is always a good option; you can't go wrong with bacon and eggs! When ordering an omelet, ask for it to be made with whole eggs. There are restaurants that actually put pancake batter in their omelets!

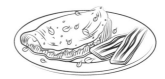

Here are some examples of foods that we often order at restaurants:

- Salad topped with protein such as salmon or steak; always request no croutons and add avocado for healthy fat

- Caesar salad, no croutons; you can add a protein

- Antipasto salad

- Bunless bacon cheeseburger; some places will wrap your burger in lettuce

- Bunless Philly cheesesteak; just about any sandwich on the menu can be ordered without a bun

- Steak with butter

- Grilled or blackened fish, no breading

- Grilled chicken, no breading

- Fajitas without the tortillas

- Taco salad without the tortilla bowl

- Burrito bowl, no rice

- Naked chicken wings with ranch or blue cheese; make sure the wings aren't breaded

- Sides such as asparagus, broccoli, Brussels sprouts, cauliflower, green beans, spaghetti squash, or zucchini noodles

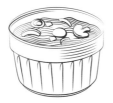

If asked, some pizzerias will make a pizza bowl with toppings only. If all else fails, you can eat the toppings and leave the crust. Use caution because it's hard to know how much sugar is in the sauce. Or you could order your pizza with no sauce or with the sauce on the side.

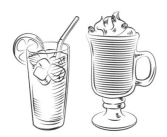

Keeping it keto at coffee shops

If you know me at all, then you know I love strong, dark coffee! The funny thing is, I didn't become a coffee drinker until my late twenties. I wonder if that has something to do with the fact that I was a busy mom of toddlers at that time? Coffee was one of the first things I knew I had to figure out for sustaining my keto life, and so many people ask me what they can drink at Starbucks. You can order a keto-friendly coffee at just about any coffee shop. There are just a few simple rules to follow:

Americano/Latte/Cappuccino— Espresso-based drinks normally have a milk base but can be made with heavy cream instead.

Brewed coffee—My easiest and favorite order is simply brewed coffee with steamed heavy cream. Asking the barista to steam the cream gives the drink a special touch. I like it so much that I sometimes steam cream for my coffee at home.

Bulletproof coffee—You've probably heard of the ever-popular bulletproof coffee, a blended drink that is usually made with butter and MCT oil. I've included a recipe on page 263. The good news is that a lot of coffee shops are getting on board with this trend. Even my local small-town coffee shop now offers bulletproof coffee.

Iced coffee or cold brew—Great ordered with a splash of heavy cream. I sometimes add a sugar-free flavored syrup.

Iced tea—A lot of coffee shops offer flavored iced teas that can be ordered unsweetened, such as peach and passionfruit.

Cream—Avoid milk; stick to heavy cream or half-and-half. Avoid coffee shop almond milk unless you can check the ingredients; shops tend to use almond milk that contains additives and sugar. I usually ask for a splash or a small amount of heavy cream so that the barista isn't too heavy-handed with it. Sometimes I bring my own cream so I know what's in it and can control the amount.

Sweeteners—Sugar-free syrups and stevia are the most popular sweetener choices. Again, you can bring your own if you like.

Snacks—Pack your own treats! Good choices from this book include Cinnamon Muffins (page 76) and Lemon Poppy Seed Loaf (page 80).

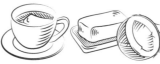

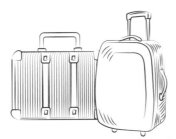

Keeping it keto while traveling

How many times have you gone on a strict diet before a vacation? How many times have you lost weight before said vacation only to go and gain it all back, plus more? I've done it countless times! I've now taken many trips and remained keto without putting on extra pounds. Whether it's a short road trip or a two-week vacation, it is possible to stay on plan and not feel deprived. I try to keep my focus on the experiences, family time, and relaxation and not the food. I'm not telling you what to do here; it's a personal choice whether or not to stay keto every single day. If you do decide to stick to the keto lifestyle when traveling, I offer you these tips:

- **Planning ahead is key!** I cannot stress this enough. Before you travel, plan as many of your meals and snacks as you can.

- **Eat foods that keep you satiated.** Protein and fat will keep you fuller longer. Try to stay away from low-carb junk food that can increase cravings.

- **Pack your own snacks, such as:**

  Beef jerky (no sugar added)　　*Nuts*

  Berries　　*Protein bars*

  Cheese

  Cut veggies

  Dark chocolate

  Nut butters

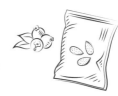

A road trip is the easiest option because it gives you the ability to pack a cooler with your favorite snacks. Traveling by air can be tricky but is definitely doable. Bring snacks that you can eat on the plane, and then buy groceries when you arrive at your destination. Scope out what is available in the area beforehand. If you won't have a car, look for Amazon Prime grocery delivery or another delivery service.

When it comes to lodgings, renting a condo or house with a full kitchen is my favorite way to vacation. With access to a kitchen, there's no reason you can't stay on plan! I get it; you're on vacation, and you don't want to cook the entire vacation. I don't like working on vacation, either. But having a kitchen makes it easier to prepare a few in-room meals.

If you must stay in a hotel, try to choose a room with a small refrigerator and microwave—even better if it has a kitchenette. If possible, choose a hotel with a full-service restaurant. This will give you more breakfast choices than a continental breakfast buffet that usually consists of waffles, cereal, and other high-carb foods.

❧ Sample Menus ❧

There's a fantastic variety of recipes in this book, so I've included some simple menus to help make putting meals together easier for you. Whether it's a special occasion or a weeknight meal with the kids, I've got you covered!

Brunch

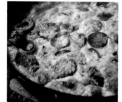
Smoked Sausage and Mushroom Breakfast Skillet *(page 56)*

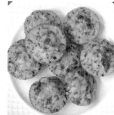
Egg Muffins *(page 66)*

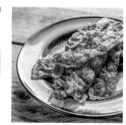
Bacon

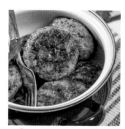
Sausage patties

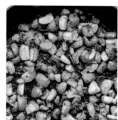
Home-Fried Bacon Radishes *(page 68)*

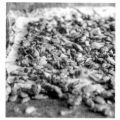

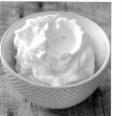
Grain-Free Granola *(page 60)* **with Whipped Cream** *(page 254)* **and assorted berries**

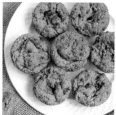
Cinnamon Muffins *(page 76)*

Fish Fry

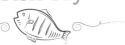

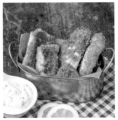 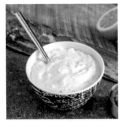 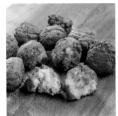

Southern Fish Fry
(page 172)

Tartar Sauce
(page 276)

Hushpuppies
(page 98)

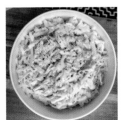 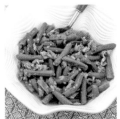 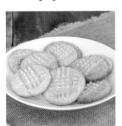

Creamy Coleslaw
(page 134)

**Old-Fashioned
Green Beans**
(page 214)

**One-Bowl
Butter Cookies**
(page 234)

Bridal Shower

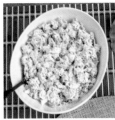 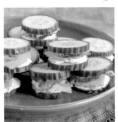 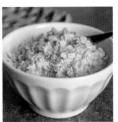 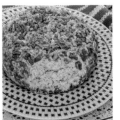

**Easy Chicken
Salad**
(page 142)

**Cucumber Finger
Sandwiches**
(page 106)

Pimento Cheese
(page 90)

**Pecan Ranch
Cheese Ball**
(page 102)

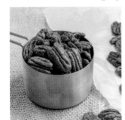 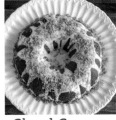 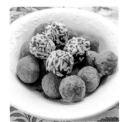

**Praline Toasted
Pecans**
(page 232)

**Glazed Coconut
Bundt Cake**
(page 248)

Easy Truffles
(page 240)

Summer Picnic

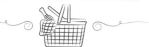

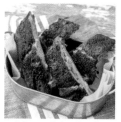 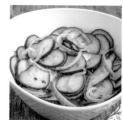 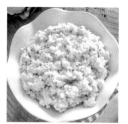 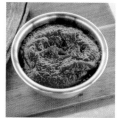

Memphis-Style Ribs
(page 152)

Easy BBQ Sauce
(page 277)

Marinated Cucumber Salad
(page 140)

Southern Fauxtato Salad
(page 136)

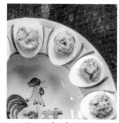 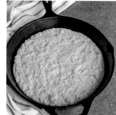 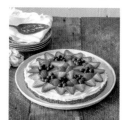

Deviled Eggs
(page 100)

Skillet Cornbread
(page 74)

Fruit Pizza
(page 226)

Football Tailgate

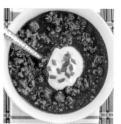 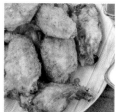 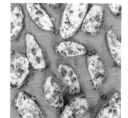

Easy Chili
(page 124)

Crispy Chicken Wings
(page 160)

Sweet Pepper Poppers
(page 96)

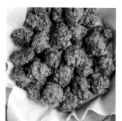 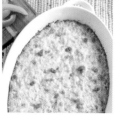 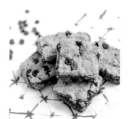

Cheesy Sausage Balls
(page 88)

Artichoke Dip
(page 86)
with veggies

Peanut Butter Chocolate Chip Cookie Bars
(page 224)

French Quarter Feast

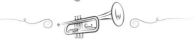

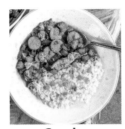 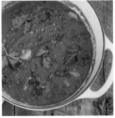 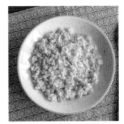

Gumbo
(page 126)

Shrimp Creole
(page 154)

Easy Cheesy
Caulirice
(page 202)

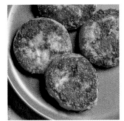 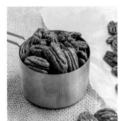

Fried Green
Tomatoes
(page 218)

Praline Toasted
Pecans
(page 232)

Thanksgiving Feast

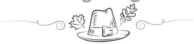

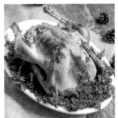 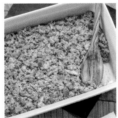 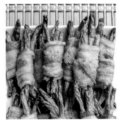 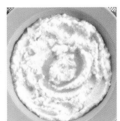

Butter Roasted
Turkey
(page 190)

Sausage Cornbread
Dressing
(page 208)

Green Bean
Bacon Bundles
(page 196)

Easy Caulimash
(page 210)

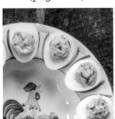 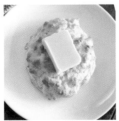 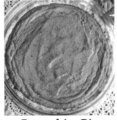 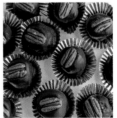

Deviled Eggs
(page 100)

Drop Biscuits
(page 72)

Pumpkin Pie
(page 250)

Kentucky
Bourbon Balls
(page 242)

Date Night

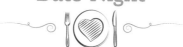

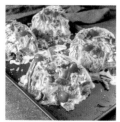 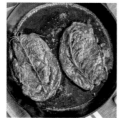 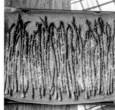 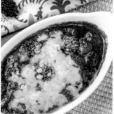

BLT Wedge Salad *(page 138)*

Reverse Sear Garlic Rosemary Rib-Eye Steaks *(page 176)*

Parmesan Asparagus *(page 211)*

Quick Blackberry Cobbler for Two *(page 238)*

Southern Supper

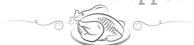

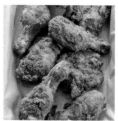 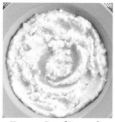 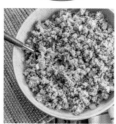 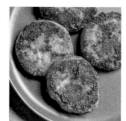 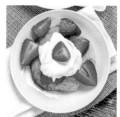

Fried Chicken *(page 182)*

Easy Caulimash *(page 210)*

Cornbread Salad *(page 144)*

Fried Green Tomatoes *(page 218)*

Strawberry Shortcakes *(page 236)*

Kid-Friendly Cuisine

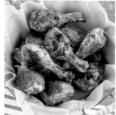 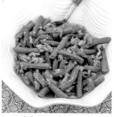 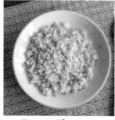 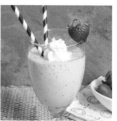

Barbecue Chicken Drumsticks *(page 174)*

Old-Fashioned Green Beans *(page 214)*

Easy Cheesy Caulirice *(page 202)*

Strawberry Milkshake *(page 258)*

❧ Recipes That Are Good for Doubling ❧

Whenever possible, I double recipes so that I have leftovers for lunches during the week. As you can see, I have listed all the soup recipes here, because in my opinion, soup always tastes better left over!

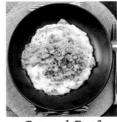

Open-Faced Sloppy Joes
(page 150)

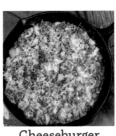

Cheeseburger "Mac" Helper
(page 162)

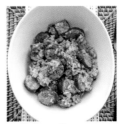

Ground Beef Stroganoff
(page 170)

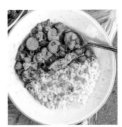

Cajun Sausage and Rice
(page 178)

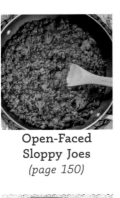

Slow Cooker Bourbon Chicken
(page 180)

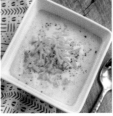

Broccoli Cheese Soup
(page 114)

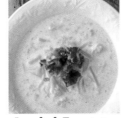

Loaded Fauxtato Soup
(page 116)

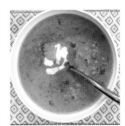

Taco Soup
(page 118)

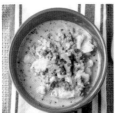

Cheeseburger Soup
(page 120)

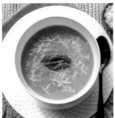

Tomato Basil Soup
(page 122)

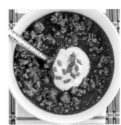

Easy Chili
(page 124)

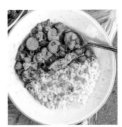

Gumbo
(page 126)

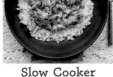
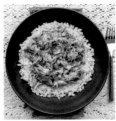

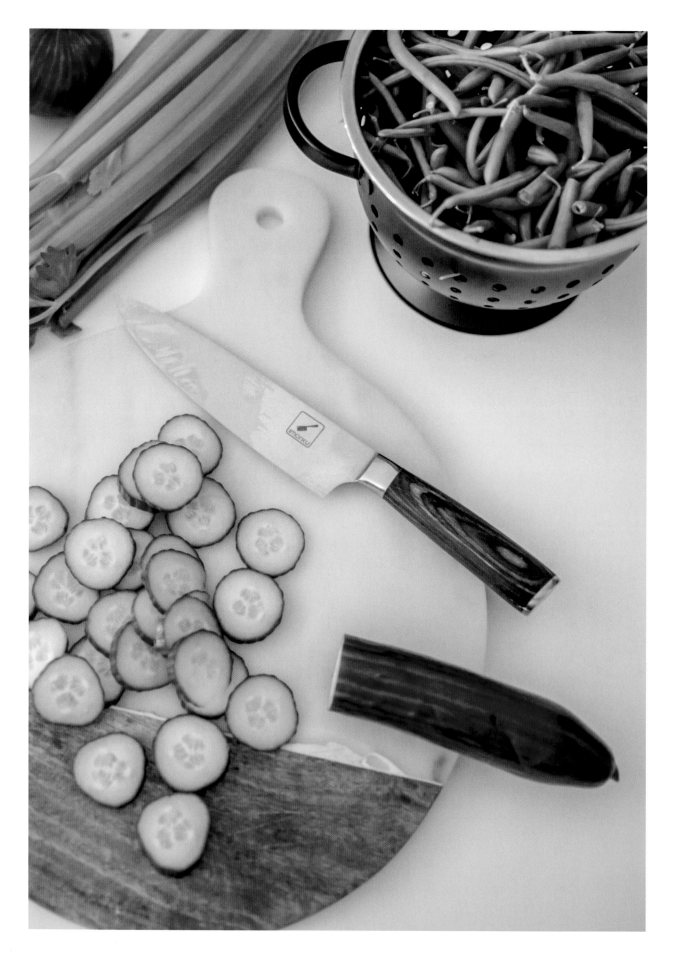

Recipes

The recipes in this book represent some of my very favorite dishes. Some are low-carb adaptations of Southern classics that I grew up eating, like Drop Biscuits with Sausage Gravy and Memphis-Style Ribs. Others are keto staples, including Deviled Eggs and Easy Caulimash. No matter where you live, I believe you'll enjoy these comforting dishes from my home to yours.

For those of you with food allergies or sensitivities, I have marked those recipes that are free of common allergens with these icons:

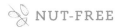 NUT-FREE

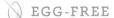 EGG-FREE

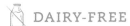 DAIRY-FREE

If an icon has the word OPTION underneath it, then the recipe can be modified to omit that allergen.

Also, I know how pressed for time we all are, so I have marked those recipes that can be made in 30 minutes or less from start to finish with this icon:

 30 MINUTES OR LESS

For a handy chart showing you which recipes fall into each of these categories, see pages 287 to 289.

NUTRITION INFORMATION is included for each recipe as well. It was calculated to the best of my ability using information from the brands of ingredients I buy. Optional ingredients are not included in these calculations. Neither is oil used for frying foods; the amount of oil absorbed cannot be calculated accurately.

I always recommend calculating your own macros; they can widely vary depending on the brands you choose. For example, different brands of cream cheese can vary by as much as 2 grams of carbs per serving. That can add up quickly! There are apps you can use, such as MyFitnessPal, to calculate macros.

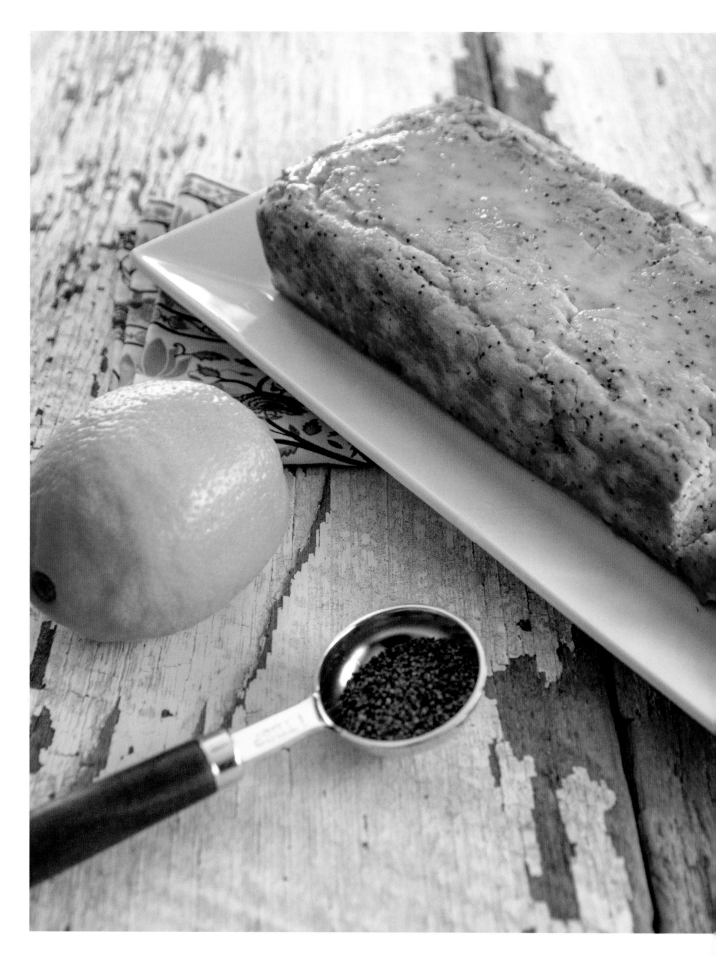

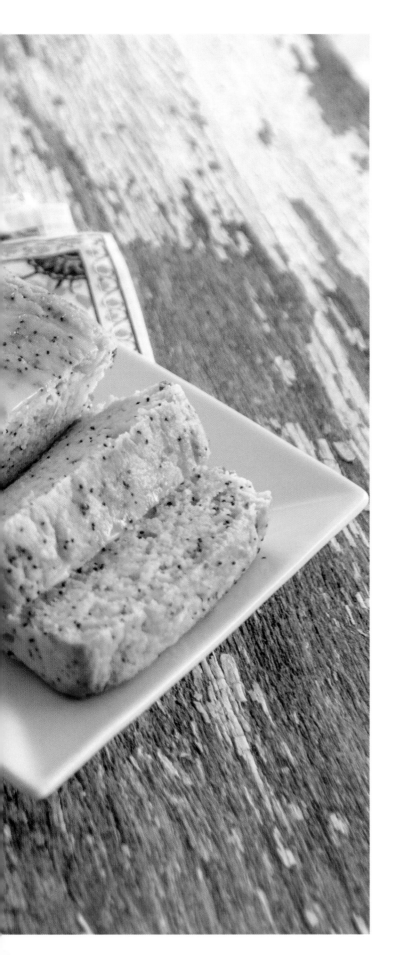

Chapter 1

Breakfast & Breads

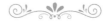

Smoked Sausage and Mushroom Breakfast Skillet

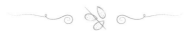

yield: 6 servings
prep time: 15 minutes
cook time: 35 minutes

This yummy breakfast skillet is easy to make and impressive to serve. Smoked sausage and eggs were made for each other! You can use any type of smoked sausage you like. I tend to use smoked beef sausage; if you want some heat, try andouille!

8 large eggs

¼ cup heavy whipping cream

1 cup shredded cheddar cheese

Pinch of salt

Pinch of ground black pepper

12 ounces smoked sausage, sliced

1 cup diced white mushrooms

¼ cup sliced green onions, plus extra for garnish if desired

1. In a medium-sized bowl, whisk together the eggs and cream, then stir in the cheese, salt, and pepper. Set aside.

2. Preheat the oven to 400°F.

3. Heat a 12-inch cast-iron skillet or other ovenproof skillet over medium heat. Cook the sausage slices until browned on both sides, 5 to 6 minutes. Add the mushrooms and green onions and continue cooking until the mushrooms are tender, about 5 minutes. Turn off the heat.

4. Pour the egg mixture evenly over the sausage and vegetables in the skillet. Bake for 25 minutes or until the eggs are set.

5. Run a knife around the edge of the skillet before slicing. Garnish with more green onions, if desired, and serve immediately. Leftovers can be stored in the refrigerator for up to 5 days. Reheat just until warmed; be careful not to overheat or the eggs will become rubbery.

NET CARBS 2.3g				
calories	fat	protein	carbs	fiber
281	22.6g	15.9g	2.6g	0.2g

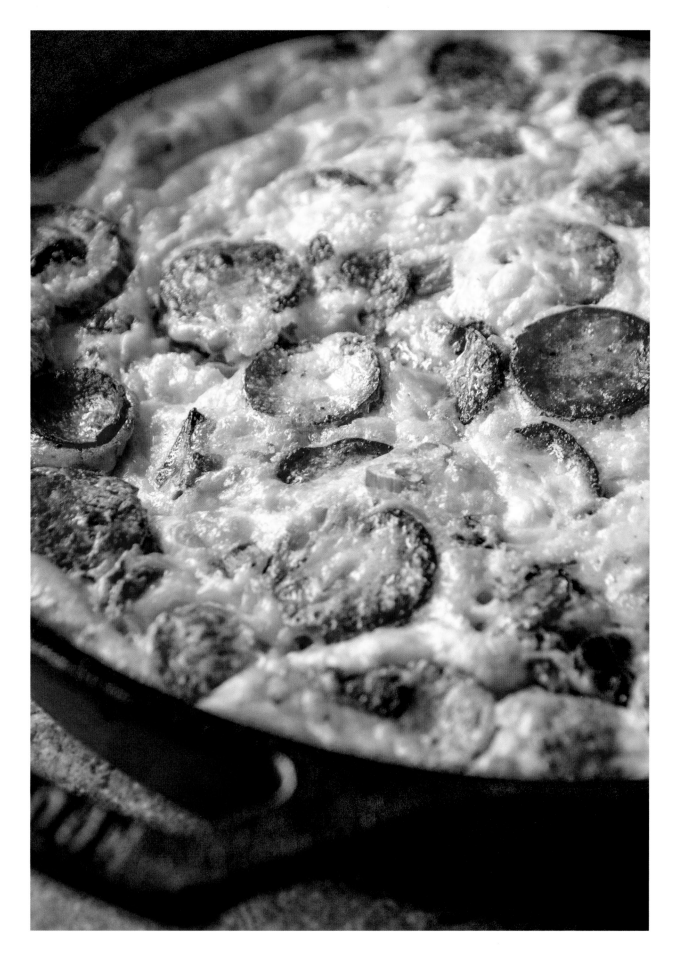

Cowboy Breakfast Skillet

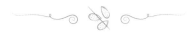

yield: 8 servings
prep time: 20 minutes
cook time: 42 minutes

A cauliflower crust adds a nice touch to this hearty breakfast skillet. It's sure to please the whole family, and they won't even suspect that there's cauliflower in it!

CRUST:

1 (12-ounce) bag frozen riced cauliflower

1 large egg

½ cup grated Parmesan cheese

¼ teaspoon salt

FILLING:

8 ounces bulk breakfast sausage

6 slices bacon, chopped

½ cup diced bell peppers (any color)

2 tablespoons chopped green onions

6 large eggs

¼ teaspoon salt

½ teaspoon ground black pepper

To make the crust:

1. Preheat the oven to 425°F. Grease a 12-inch cast-iron skillet or other ovenproof skillet with oil.

2. Cook the cauliflower according to the package directions. Allow to cool slightly, then use cheesecloth or paper towels to absorb any excess water.

3. In a medium-sized bowl, mix together the cooked cauliflower, egg, Parmesan cheese, and salt. Press the mixture evenly across the bottom of the prepared skillet. Par-bake the crust for 12 minutes or until it starts to brown around the edges, then remove from the oven and set aside to cool. Leave the oven on. While the crust is baking, make the filling.

To make the filling:

1. In a skillet over medium heat, cook the sausage, bacon, bell peppers, and green onions, crumbling the sausage with a large spoon as it cooks, until the meats are fully cooked and the vegetables are tender, about 10 minutes. Remove from the heat and set aside.

2. In a medium-sized bowl, whisk together the eggs, salt, and pepper. Add the meat mixture to the eggs and stir until well combined.

3. Pour the filling over the cooled, par-baked crust and spread evenly.

4. Return the skillet to the oven and bake for 20 minutes or until the eggs are set and slightly firm to the touch. Run a knife around the edge of the skillet before slicing. Serve immediately. Leftovers can be stored in the refrigerator for up to 5 days. Reheat just until warmed; be careful not to overheat or the eggs will become rubbery.

NET CARBS 3.3g				
calories	fat	protein	carbs	fiber
338	26g	19.7g	5.8g	2.5g

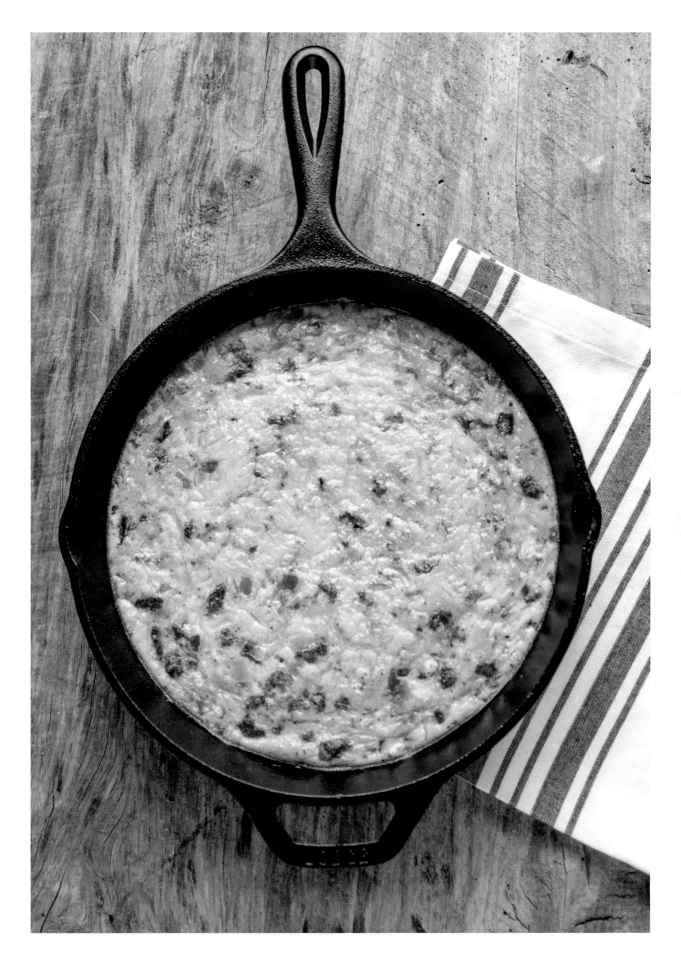

Grain-Free Granola

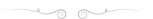

yield: 3 cups (¼ cup per serving)

prep time: 5 minutes

cook time: 30 minutes

I've always loved snacking on granola, and back in the day I was one to enjoy the occasional bowl of cereal for breakfast. My grain-free granola fits the bill for both! When I eat it with unsweetened almond milk, it really satisfies my craving for cereal. The pecans and coconut chips add just the right Southern touch.

1 cup chopped raw pecans

1 cup roasted and salted shelled sunflower seeds

1 cup unsweetened coconut flakes

¼ cup finely ground blanched almond flour

1 large egg white

¼ cup granular erythritol

2 tablespoons salted butter, melted

1 teaspoon vanilla extract

⅛ teaspoon liquid stevia

1. Preheat the oven to 325°F. Line a sheet pan with parchment paper.

2. In a medium-sized bowl, stir together the pecans, sunflower seeds, coconut flakes, and almond flour.

3. In a small bowl, whisk the egg white, then stir in the erythritol, melted butter, vanilla extract, and stevia. Pour over the pecan mixture and stir until the pecan mixture is completely coated with the egg white mixture.

4. Spread the granola evenly on the sheet pan. Bake for 25 to 30 minutes, stirring every 10 minutes, until light golden brown. Allow to cool completely before serving. Leftovers can be stored in an airtight container for up to 2 weeks.

NET CARBS 1.6g				
calories	fat	protein	carbs	fiber
186	18.1g	4g	4.5g	2.9g

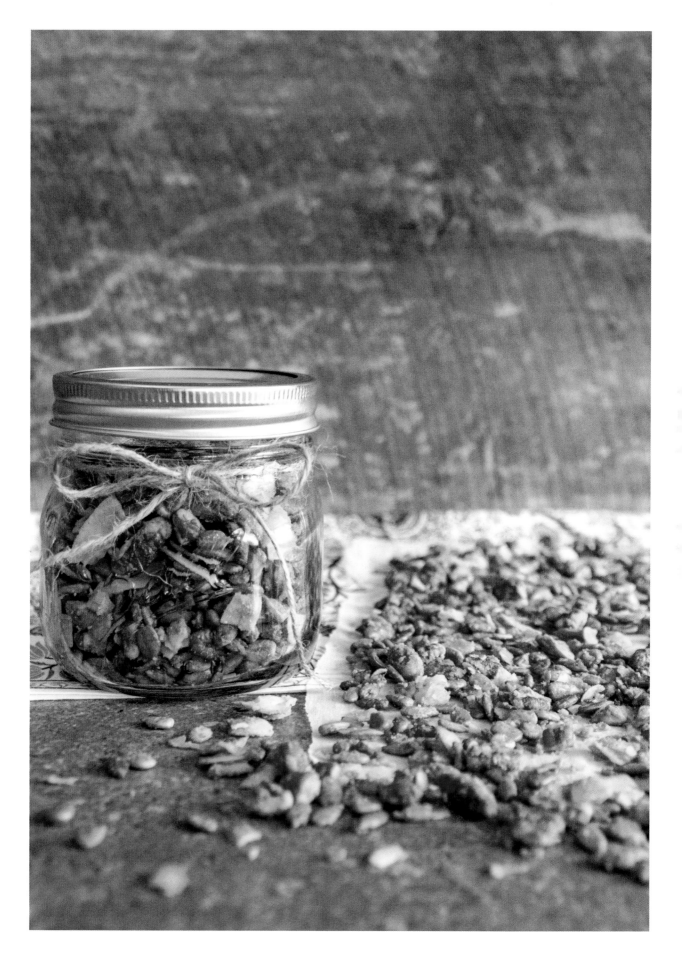

Skillet Pancake Puff

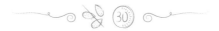

yield: 4 servings
prep time: 5 minutes
cook time: 20 minutes

Pancakes are a popular Southern breakfast comfort food; in fact, there's a pancake house on nearly every corner in the Smoky Mountains of Tennessee. Since going keto, though, I can't simply run down to the local pancake house to get my fill. And sometimes I want pancakes but I don't want to go to the trouble to cook up batch after batch. This large skillet pancake is the answer—it's both easy and delicious.

2 tablespoons salted butter

4 large eggs

¼ cup water

¼ cup heavy whipping cream

2 tablespoons coconut flour

2 tablespoons granular erythritol

½ teaspoon vanilla extract

¼ teaspoon salt

FOR GARNISH (optional):

Fresh blueberries

Confectioners'-style erythritol

1. Preheat the oven to 425°F.

2. Put the butter in a 10-inch cast-iron skillet or other ovenproof skillet and place it in the oven to melt the butter. When the butter is melted, remove the skillet from the oven.

3. In a medium-sized bowl, whisk the eggs. Using a spoon, mix in the water, cream, coconut flour, erythritol, vanilla extract, and salt. Continue stirring until the batter is well blended.

4. Pour the batter into the hot skillet and bake for 18 to 20 minutes, until the pancake is puffed and golden. Slice into quarters and garnish with blueberries and confectioners'-style erythritol, if desired.

NET CARBS 1g				
calories	fat	protein	carbs	fiber
164	13.8g	7.2g	1.7g	0.7g

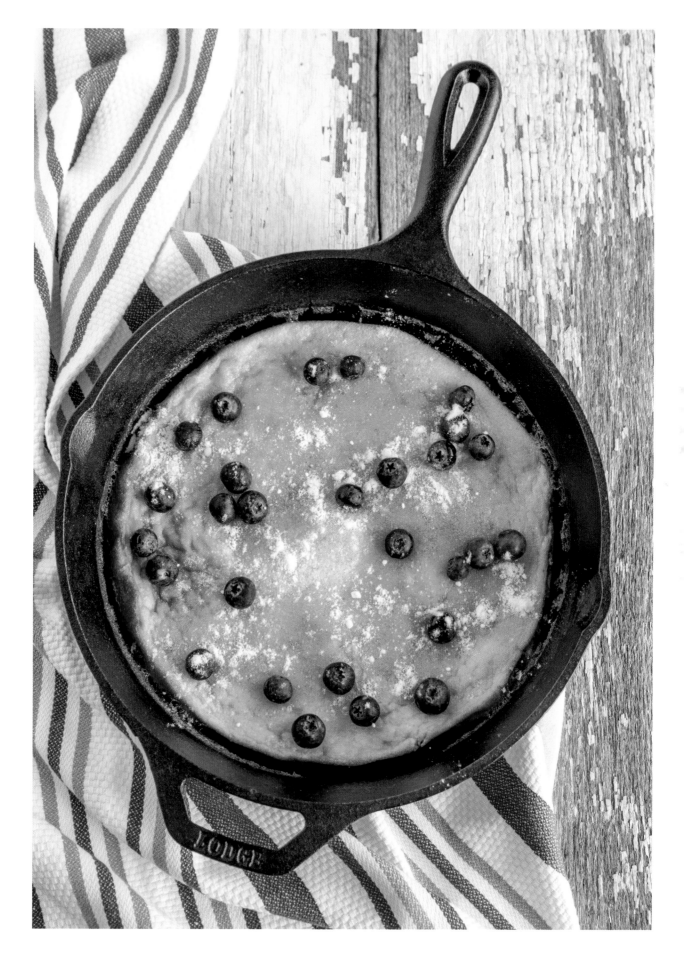

Waffles

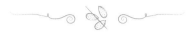

yield: 6 waffles (2 per serving)
prep time: 5 minutes
cook time: 30 minutes

Who says you have to give up waffles on a keto diet? These are so much better than those frozen boxed waffles I ate as a child. I didn't even own a waffle maker before I went keto. I decided to get one because I wanted more breakfast choices. I have never regretted that purchase. These waffles are delicious and easy to make. You can make extras and eat them all week!

1 (8-ounce) package cream cheese, cubed

6 large eggs

2 tablespoons granular erythritol

1 tablespoon baking powder

2 teaspoons ground cinnamon

1 teaspoon vanilla extract

Pinch of salt

SERVING SUGGESTIONS:

Sugar-free pancake syrup

Fresh blueberries

Butter

1. Preheat a waffle iron according to the manufacturer's directions.

2. Place all the ingredients in a blender and blend until very smooth. Allow the batter to rest for 10 minutes.

3. Grease the hot waffle iron with oil. Pour enough of the batter into the waffle iron to make one waffle. (Check the manufacturer's instructions for the exact amount of batter to use.) Be careful to not overfill the waffle iron because these waffles will expand; if you overfill the iron, the batter will overflow. Cook the waffle until it's golden brown.

4. Carefully remove the waffle and repeat the cooking process with the rest of the batter. Serve with syrup, blueberries, and/or butter, if desired. Leftovers can be stored in an airtight container in the refrigerator for up to 5 days. Reheat in the toaster.

SPECIAL EQUIPMENT:

Waffle iron

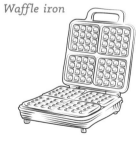

Notes:
Omit the sweetener and vanilla extract to make savory waffles for sandwiches!

This batter can also be used to make pancakes, but we like it better as waffles.

NET CARBS 2.6g				
calories	fat	protein	carbs	fiber
343	25.7g	18g	3.5g	0.9g

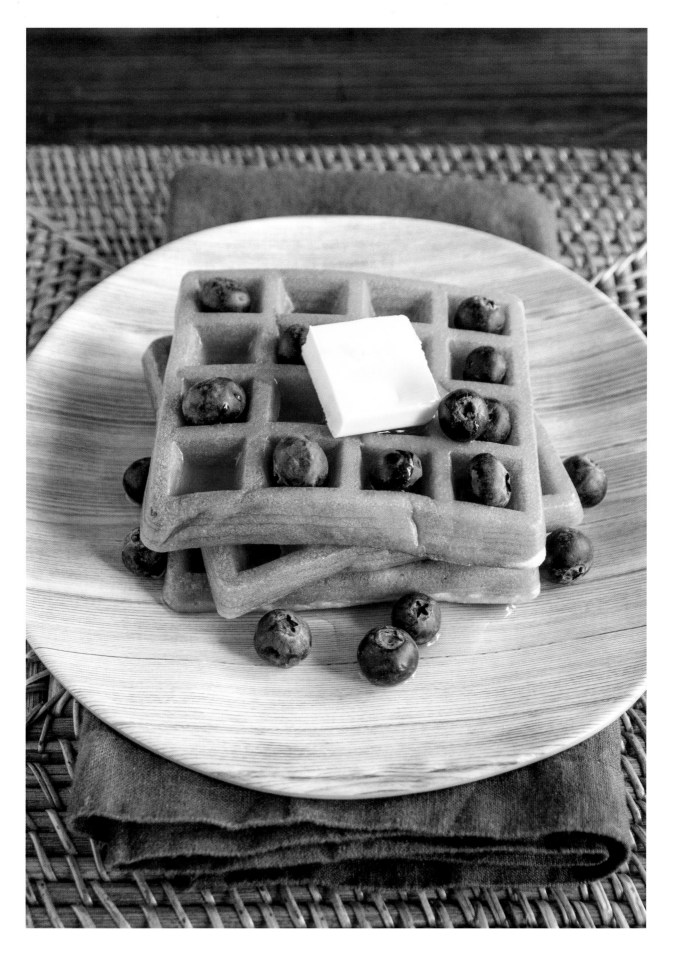

Egg Muffins

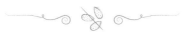

yield: 10 muffins (1 per serving)

prep time: 5 minutes

cook time: 30 minutes

8 ounces bulk breakfast sausage

2 teaspoons dried chives

6 large eggs

¼ cup heavy whipping cream

1 teaspoon dried ground oregano

¼ teaspoon salt

½ teaspoon pepper

¾ cup shredded sharp cheddar cheese

Egg muffins are popular everywhere now, including the South, because everyone needs a quick but wholesome breakfast option. They are so simple to make, and they reheat nicely, which makes them perfect for those busy weekday mornings!

1. Preheat the oven to 350°F. Grease 10 wells of a standard-size 12-well muffin pan with oil.

2. In a medium-sized skillet over medium heat, cook the sausage with the chives, crumbling the meat with a large spoon as it cooks, until the sausage is well browned and cooked through, about 10 minutes. Drain the fat, if necessary, and set aside.

3. Whisk the eggs in a medium-sized bowl, then add the cream, oregano, salt, and pepper and whisk until well combined. Stir in the cooked sausage mixture and the cheese.

4. Pour the mixture into the prepared wells of the muffin pan, filling each well about three-quarters full.

5. Bake the muffins for 15 to 20 minutes, until the centers are set and the tops are lightly browned. Leftovers can be stored in an airtight container in the refrigerator for up to a week. Reheat just until warmed; be careful not to overheat or the eggs will become rubbery.

NET CARBS 0.6g				
calories	fat	protein	carbs	fiber
165	13.7g	9.1g	0.7g	0.1g

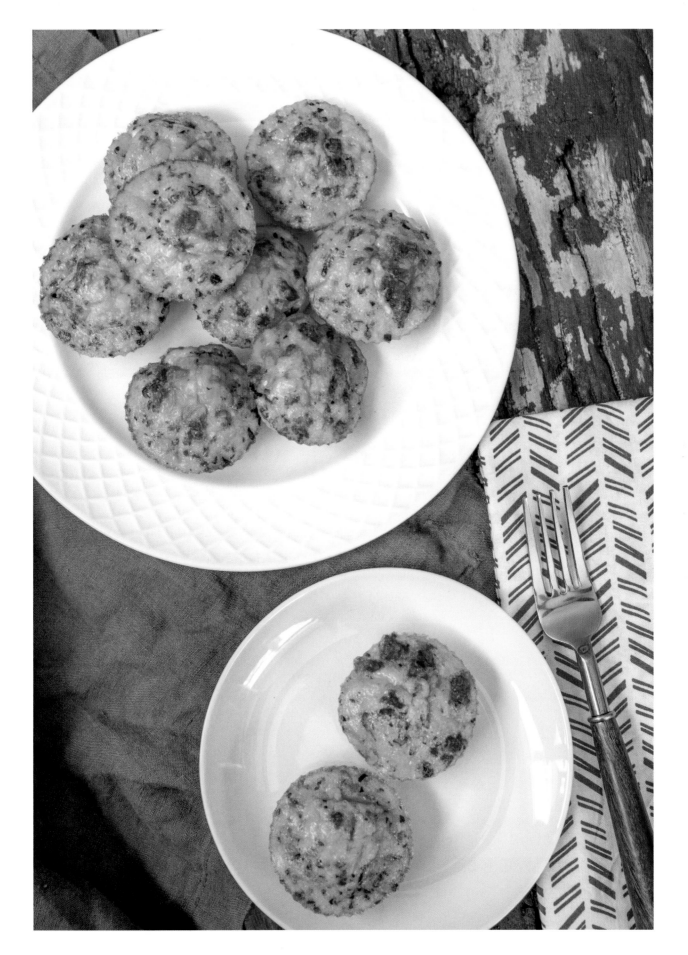

Home-Fried Bacon Radishes

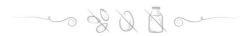

yield: 4 servings

prep time: 10 minutes

cook time: 25 minutes

Growing up, my mom frequently made me fried potatoes. These radishes remind me of fried potatoes! This versatile dish can be served with breakfast (for example, in place of hash browns) or dinner.

1 (16-ounce) bag radishes

6 slices bacon

Salt and ground black pepper

Chopped fresh flat-leaf parsley, for garnish (optional)

1. Trim the tops off the radishes and chop the radishes into small pieces.

2. In a large skillet over medium heat, cook the bacon until crispy, about 5 minutes. Remove the bacon from the skillet, leaving the drippings in the pan. Crumble the bacon and set aside.

3. Place the radishes in the skillet and cook over medium-high heat for 10 minutes, then reduce the heat to medium. Add the cooked bacon and continue cooking for about 10 more minutes, stirring every couple of minutes, until the radishes are slightly crispy and caramelized around the edges.

4. Season to taste with salt and pepper and serve immediately. Garnish with parsley, if desired.

NET CARBS 2g				
calories	fat	protein	carbs	fiber
100	6.9g	6g	3.9g	1.8g

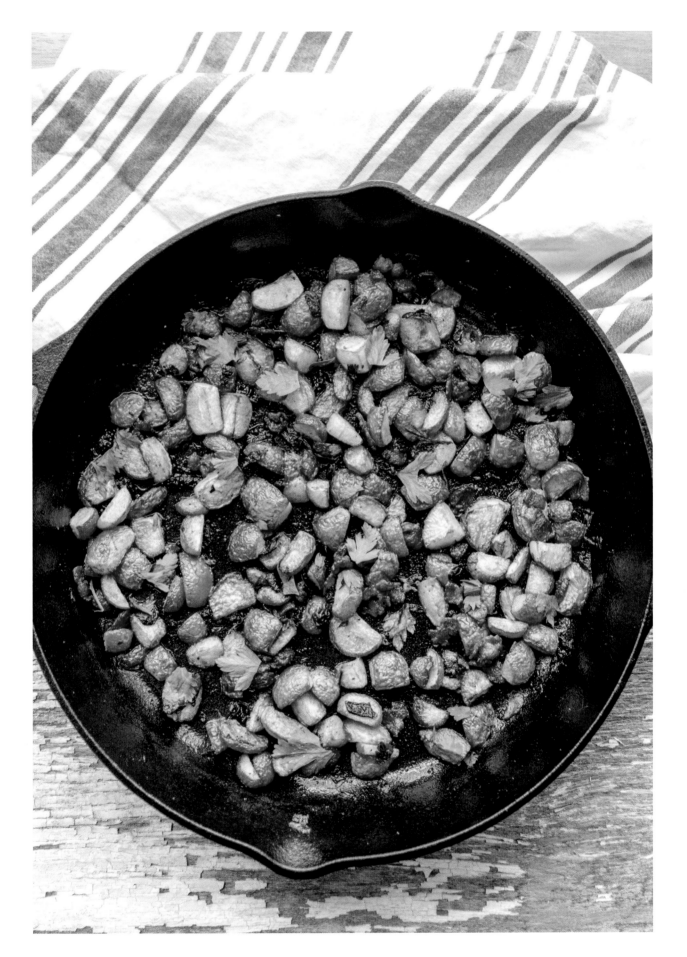

Sausage Gravy

OPTION

yield: 6 servings (½ cup per serving)

prep time: 5 minutes

cook time: 20 minutes

This sausage gravy is the perfect accompaniment to my Drop Biscuits. I developed the two recipes to satisfy my urge for biscuits and gravy, a classic dish that you can find on just about every restaurant menu in the South. In my high-carb days, it was my favorite breakfast to order at a restaurant. This gravy also is great served over scrambled eggs, for those days when you don't feel like making biscuits, or if you want a nut-free breakfast.

1 pound bulk breakfast sausage

1 cup heavy whipping cream

¾ cup water

½ teaspoon xanthan gum

Salt and ground black pepper

6 Drop Biscuits (page 72), for serving (optional)

1. In a large skillet over medium heat, cook the sausage, crumbling the meat with a large spoon as it cooks, until it is well browned, about 10 minutes.

2. Reduce the heat to low. Stir in the cream, water, and xanthan gum. Continue cooking, stirring frequently, until the gravy starts to thicken, about 10 minutes. If it gets too thick, thin it with water, adding a tablespoon at a time.

3. Season the gravy to taste with salt and pepper. Serve over biscuits, if desired. The gravy is best served right away, but leftovers can be stored in the refrigerator for up to 5 days.

NET CARBS 1.5g				
calories	fat	protein	carbs	fiber
199	18.4g	9g	1.6g	0.2g

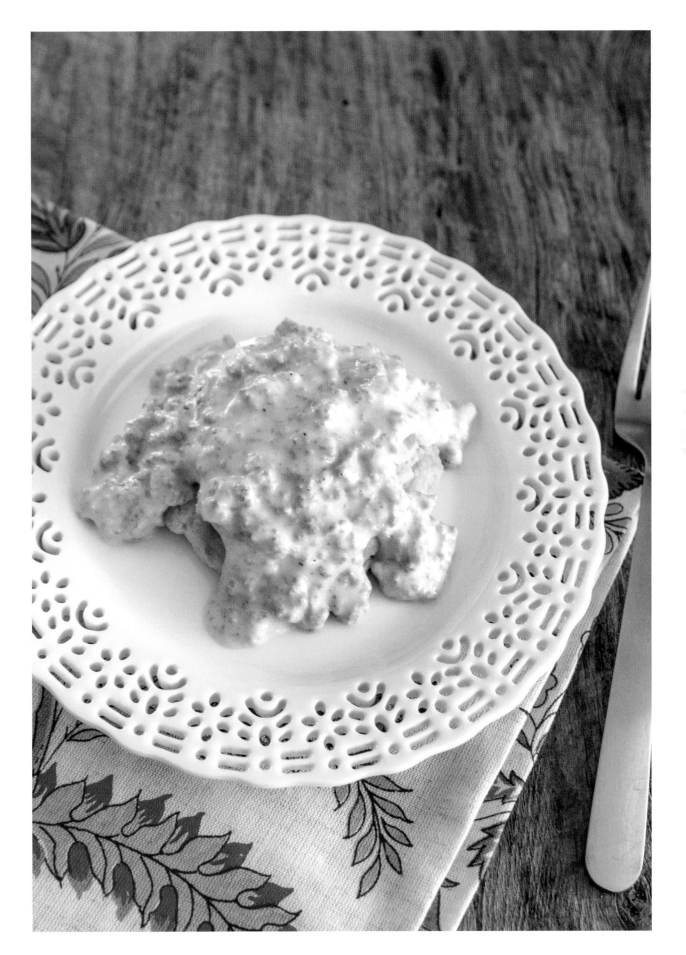

Drop Biscuits

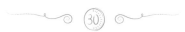

yield: 10 biscuits (1 per serving)

prep time: 10 minutes

cook time: 12 minutes

When I was a little girl, I spent a lot of time with my Great-Aunt Nannie. Every morning, she made homemade biscuits, and she taught me how to make them. I've always loved homemade biscuits, and these keto drop biscuits are a good substitute. They are wonderful topped with a pat of butter or some Sausage Gravy (page 70). I've also included a variation that makes them taste a lot like those tasty little cheddar biscuits that Red Lobster serves!

1½ cups finely ground blanched almond flour

2 teaspoons baking powder

¼ teaspoon salt

¼ cup sour cream

2 large eggs

2 tablespoons salted butter, melted but not hot

1. Preheat the oven to 400°F. Grease a baking sheet with oil or line it with parchment paper.

2. In a medium-sized bowl, whisk together the almond flour, baking powder, and salt.

3. In a small bowl, whisk together the sour cream, eggs, and melted butter. Pour the wet mixture into the dry ingredients and stir until well combined. Allow the batter to sit for 5 minutes.

4. Drop the batter by the large spoonful onto the prepared baking sheet, leaving about 2 inches between the biscuits. Bake for 10 to 12 minutes, until the tops are golden brown. Allow to cool before removing from the pan. Leftovers can be stored in an airtight container in the refrigerator for up to a week. The biscuits can be reheated in the microwave for a few seconds; be careful not to overheat.

Variation:
Garlic Cheddar Biscuits. To the dry ingredients in Step 2, add 1 cup shredded sharp cheddar cheese, 1 teaspoon dried or fresh chives, and ½ teaspoon garlic powder.

NET CARBS 1.5g				
calories	fat	protein	carbs	fiber
142	12.1g	4.6g	3.1g	1.6g

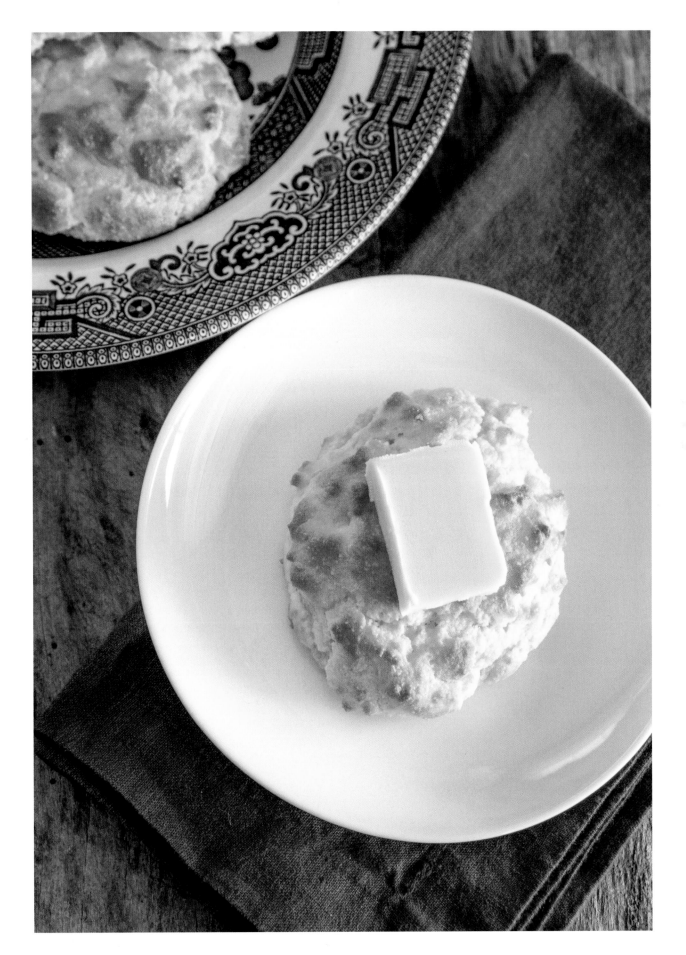

Skillet Cornbread

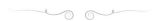

yield: 10 servings
prep time: 10 minutes
cook time: 30 minutes

Cornbread was a staple in my Grandma Ida Mae's house when I was growing up; I believe she made it every day. In the evenings, Papa would eat the leftovers as a snack crumbled up in a glass of cold buttermilk. It's hard to measure up to Grandma's cornbread, but this keto-friendly recipe is a great substitute for the high-carb version.

5 tablespoons salted butter, divided

3 large eggs

¼ cup heavy whipping cream

2 tablespoons water

2 cups finely ground blanched almond flour

2 tablespoons golden flaxseed meal

2 teaspoons baking powder

½ teaspoon salt

½ teaspoon sweet corn extract (optional) (see Note)

1. Preheat the oven to 375°F.

2. Put 2 tablespoons of the butter in a 10-inch cast-iron skillet or other ovenproof skillet and place it in the oven to melt the butter. Either in the microwave or in a small saucepan on the stovetop, heat the remaining 3 tablespoons of butter just until melted.

3. In a medium-sized bowl, whisk together the eggs, cream, water, and 3 tablespoons of melted butter.

4. In a small bowl, whisk together the almond flour, flaxseed meal, baking powder, and salt. Stir the flour mixture into the egg mixture until well combined. Stir in the corn extract, if using.

5. Pour the batter into the prepared skillet and bake for 25 to 30 minutes, until lightly browned on top and around the edges. Leftovers can be stored in a covered container in the refrigerator for up to 5 days.

Note:
The sweet corn extract is not required but is recommended for a fuller cornbread flavor.

NET CARBS 2.1g				
calories	fat	protein	carbs	fiber
233	20.6g	7g	4.6g	2.6g

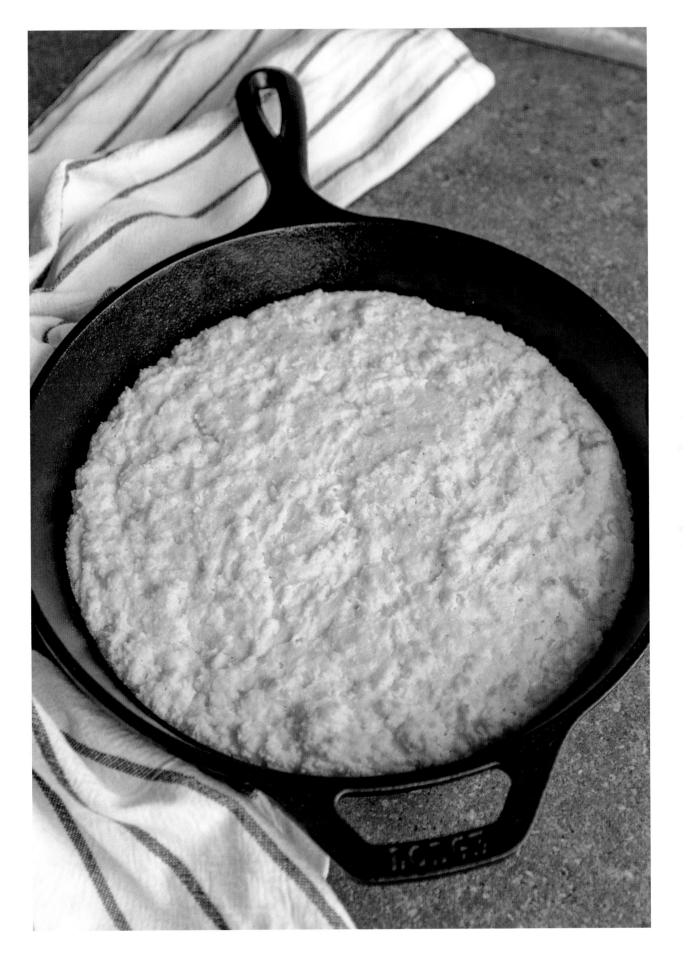

Cinnamon Muffins

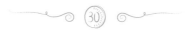

yield: 12 muffins (2 per serving)

prep time: 10 minutes

cook time: 14 minutes

In the South, we love any and all muffins, sweet and savory. These muffins remind me a bit of coffee cake. They are delicious and so easy to make. They are great for breakfast on the go and would even make a nice dessert with a fresh cup of coffee.

1½ cups finely ground blanched almond flour

1 tablespoon baking powder

1 tablespoon plus 1 teaspoon ground cinnamon, divided

2 large eggs

½ cup granular erythritol

2 tablespoons salted butter, softened

1 tablespoon heavy whipping cream

½ teaspoon vanilla extract

⅛ teaspoon liquid stevia

1. Preheat the oven to 350°F. Grease a standard-size 12-well muffin pan.

2. In a small bowl, whisk together the almond flour, baking powder, and 1 tablespoon of the cinnamon; set aside.

3. In a medium-sized bowl, whisk the eggs, then add the erythritol, butter, cream, vanilla extract, stevia, and remaining 1 teaspoon of cinnamon and stir until the ingredients are well combined. Slowly add the flour mixture, stirring with a spoon until the batter is smooth.

4. Pour the batter into the prepared muffin pan, filling each well about three-quarters full. Bake for 12 to 14 minutes, until a toothpick or tester inserted in the middle of a muffin comes out clean.

5. Allow the muffins to cool completely before removing from the pan. Leftovers can be stored in an airtight container at room temperature for up to 3 days or in the refrigerator for up to a week.

Note:

Using silicone muffin cups is my favorite way to ensure that these muffins don't stick.

NET CARBS 2.9g				
calories	fat	protein	carbs	fiber
218	19.2g	7.4g	6.3g	3.4g

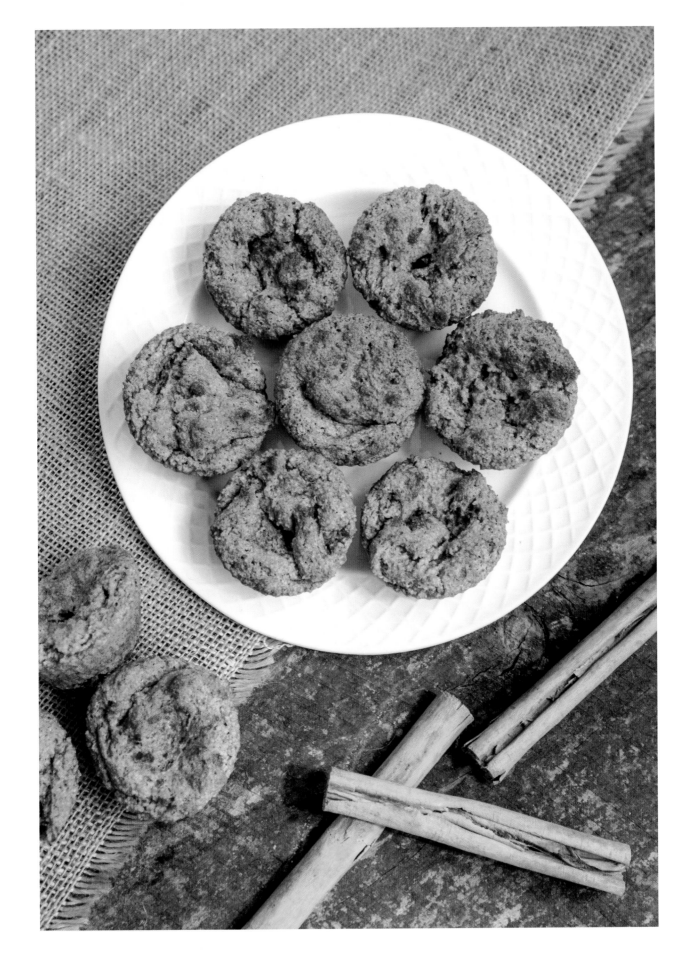

Blueberry Muffins

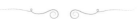

yield: 12 muffins (2 per serving)

prep time: 10 minutes

cook time: 30 minutes

I used to buy those little packages of Martha White muffin mix. We thought we loved them, but this keto version beats those muffins by a mile! This recipe keeps the carbs low by using only a half cup of blueberries, but these muffins taste just right.

1½ cups finely ground blanched almond flour

½ cup granular erythritol

2 teaspoons baking powder

¼ teaspoon salt

2 large eggs

¼ cup sour cream

½ teaspoon vanilla extract

½ cup fresh blueberries

1. Preheat the oven to 350°F. Grease a standard-size 12-well muffin pan.

2. In a small bowl, whisk together the almond flour, erythritol, baking powder, and salt.

3. In a medium-sized bowl, whisk the eggs, then stir in the sour cream and vanilla extract. Slowly add the flour mixture, stirring until well blended. Gently stir in the blueberries.

4. Pour the batter into the prepared muffin pan, filling each well about three-quarters full. Bake for 25 to 30 minutes, until the tops are lightly browned and a toothpick or tester inserted in the middle of a muffin comes out clean.

5. Allow the muffins to cool completely before removing from the pan. Leftovers can be stored in an airtight container at room temperature for up to 3 days or in the refrigerator for up to a week.

Note:
Using silicone muffin cups is my favorite way to ensure that these muffins don't stick.

NET CARBS 3.8g				
calories	fat	protein	carbs	fiber
193	14.8g	7.3g	6.6g	2.8g

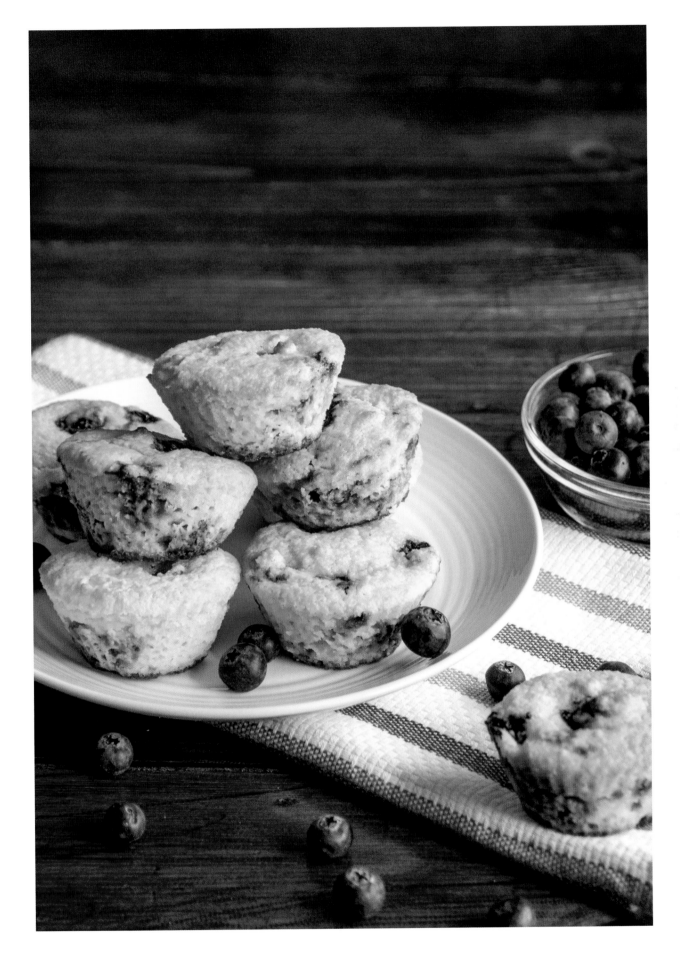

Lemon Poppy Seed Loaf

yield: 8 servings
prep time: 15 minutes
cook time: 1 hour

Southerners love lemony desserts. My husband is no exception. He loves those lemon loaf slices from Starbucks, but they are loaded with sugar and carbs! This loaf is my alternative, with the addition of poppy seeds. Here's an idea: Make a loaf of this bread and pack your own slice to take to your favorite coffee shop. Buy your coffee there, of course.

½ cup coconut flour

½ cup granular erythritol

2 teaspoons baking powder

¼ teaspoon xanthan gum

¼ teaspoon salt

3 large eggs

½ cup sour cream

1 tablespoon avocado oil

½ teaspoon vanilla extract

1 tablespoon poppy seeds

Grated zest and juice of 1 lemon

GLAZE (optional):

¼ cup heavy whipping cream

¼ cup confectioners'-style erythritol

1. Preheat the oven to 325°F. Line a 9 by 5-inch loaf pan with parchment paper or grease the pan with oil.

2. In a small bowl, whisk together the coconut flour, erythritol, baking powder, xanthan gum, and salt.

3. In a larger bowl, whisk the eggs, then add the sour cream, oil, and vanilla extract and whisk until blended. Slowly stir the flour mixture into the egg mixture with a spoon until the batter is well combined. Stir in the poppy seeds, lemon zest, and lemon juice.

4. Pour the batter into the prepared loaf pan and bake for 50 to 60 minutes, until the loaf is golden brown on top and a toothpick or tester inserted in the middle comes out clean.

5. While the loaf is baking, make the glaze, if desired: Mix the cream and erythritol in a small bowl until the sweetener is fully dissolved and the glaze is smooth; set aside.

6. As soon as you remove the loaf from the oven, spread the glaze evenly over the top. Allow the loaf to cool completely before removing from the pan and slicing. Leftovers can be stored in an airtight container at room temperature for up to 3 days or in the refrigerator for up to a week.

NET CARBS 1.9g				
calories	fat	protein	carbs	fiber
88	5.8g	4g	3.8g	1.9g

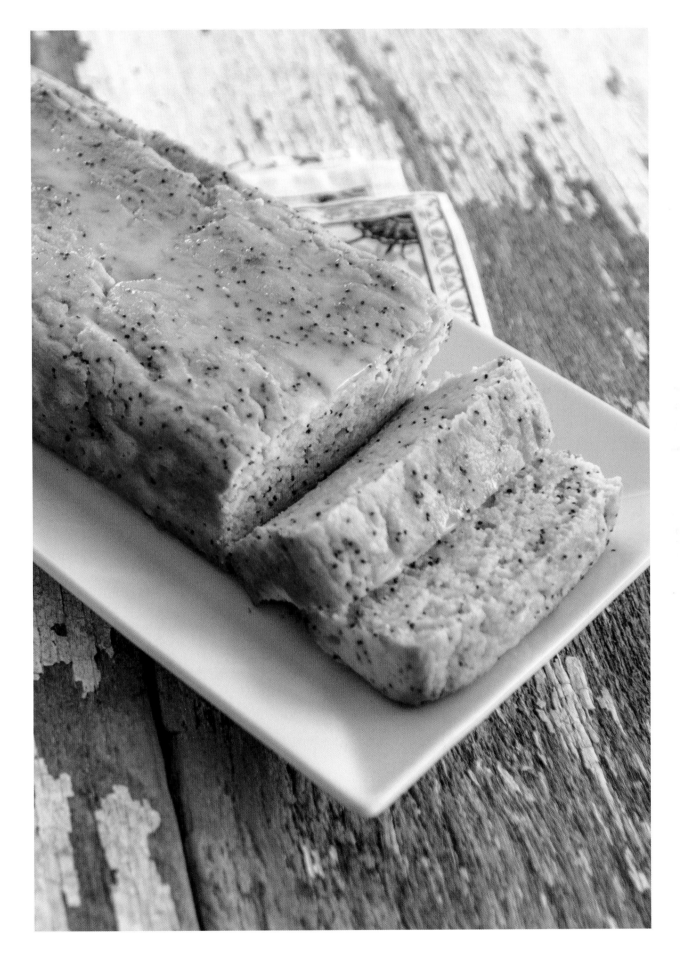

Zucchini Bread

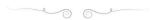

yield: 8 servings
prep time: 20 minutes
cook time: 45 minutes

Zucchini is one of those vegetables that's always plentiful in backyard gardens in the South. Everyone searches for ways to use up that zucchini. Well, here you are! What better way to use up your vegetables than in a sweet treat?

1½ cups finely ground blanched almond flour

¼ cup oat fiber

½ teaspoon baking powder

½ teaspoon baking soda

1 teaspoon ground cinnamon

½ teaspoon ginger powder

½ teaspoon ground nutmeg

½ teaspoon salt

3 large eggs

¼ cup (½ stick) salted butter, softened

½ cup granular erythritol

1 cup shredded zucchini

1. Preheat the oven to 325°F. Line a 9 by 5-inch loaf pan with parchment paper or grease the pan with oil.

2. In a medium-sized bowl, stir together the almond flour, oat fiber, baking powder, baking soda, cinnamon, ginger, nutmeg, and salt.

3. In a large bowl, use a hand mixer on low speed to beat the eggs, butter, and erythritol until well blended. With the mixer still on low speed, slowly blend in the flour mixture. Use a spoon to gently stir in the zucchini until completely combined.

4. Pour the batter into the prepared pan. Bake for 45 minutes or until the bread is lightly browned on top and a toothpick or tester inserted in the middle comes out clean.

5. Let cool in the pan for 10 minutes, then remove from the pan and allow to cool completely before slicing and serving. Leftovers can be stored in an airtight container in the refrigerator for up to 5 days.

NET CARBS 2.7g				
calories	fat	protein	carbs	fiber
267	22.8g	8.6g	11.2g	8.5g

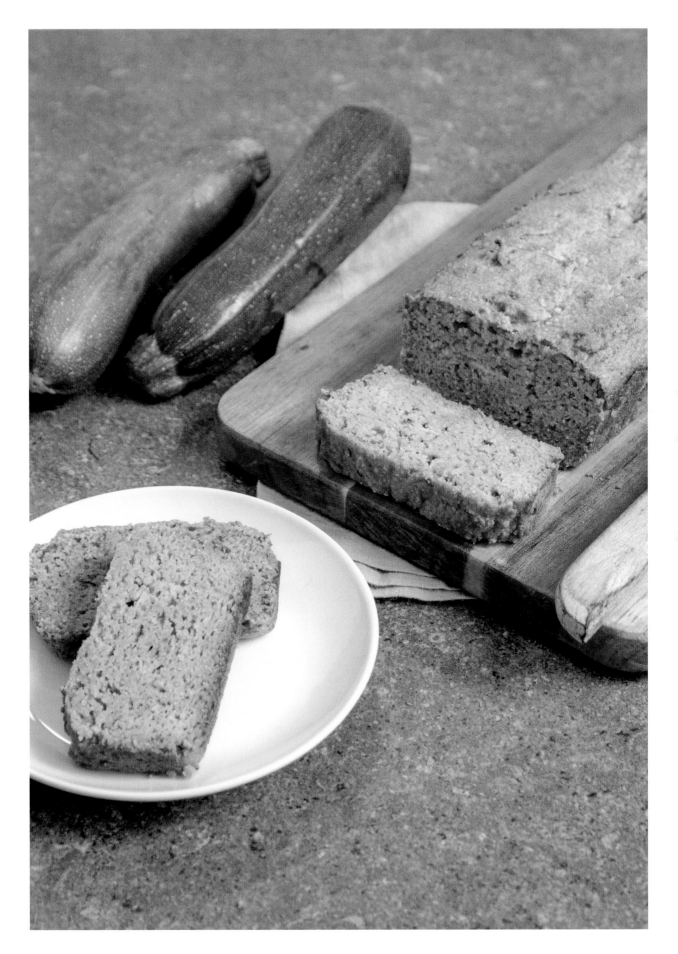

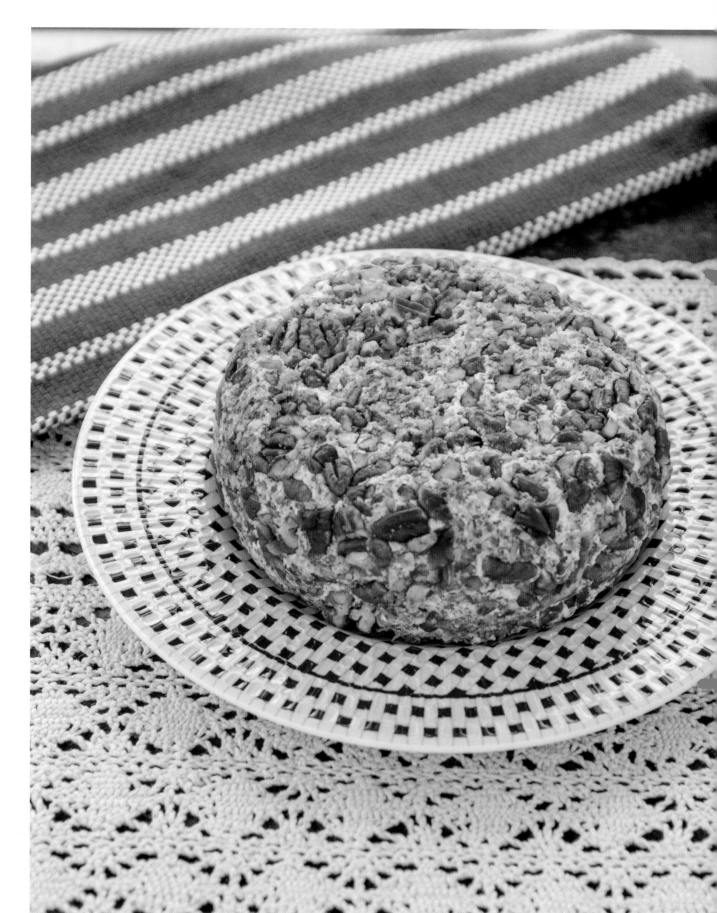

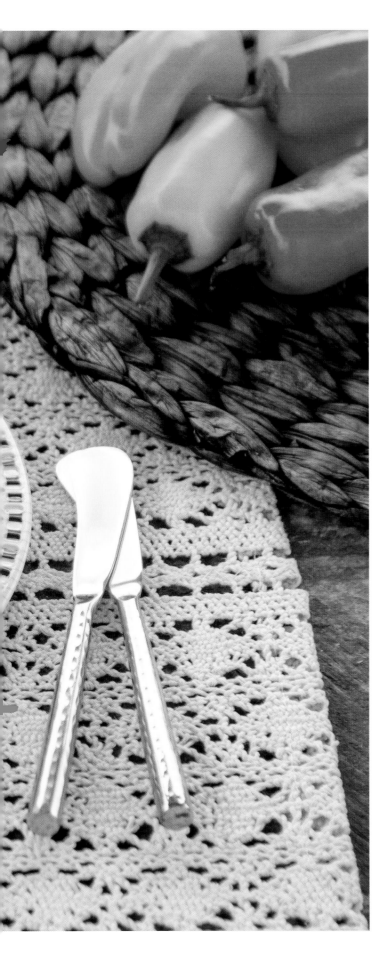

Appetizers & Snacks

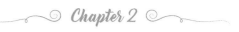

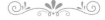

Artichoke Dip

yield: 8 servings

prep time: 10 minutes

cook time: 30 minutes

Artichoke dip is something my family has loved for years. I often make it for football parties. I'm so glad it's keto when you cut out the chips. And the perfect keto chip replacement happens to be an all-time favorite Southern snack: pork rinds! Sliced veggies and Cheese Crisps are two other great dippers.

1 (14-ounce) can quartered artichoke hearts, finely chopped

1 (8-ounce) package cream cheese, softened

1 cup mayonnaise

1 cup shredded mozzarella cheese

½ cup grated Parmesan cheese

2 cloves garlic, minced

1 green onion, finely chopped

¼ teaspoon ground black pepper

Sliced green onions, for garnish (optional)

SERVING SUGGESTIONS:

Cheese Crisps (page 94)

Sliced bell peppers, cucumbers, or other veggies

Pork rinds

1. Preheat the oven to 375°F. Grease a 9 by 13-inch baking dish.

2. In a medium-sized bowl, stir together all the ingredients until well combined.

3. Spread the dip evenly in the greased baking dish. Bake for 25 to 30 minutes, until the dip is bubbling around the edges and browned on top. Garnish with sliced green onions, if desired, and serve with the dippers of your choice. Leftovers can be stored in an airtight container in the refrigerator for up to a week.

NET CARBS 3.1g				
calories	fat	protein	carbs	fiber
372	34g	9.9g	4g	0.8g

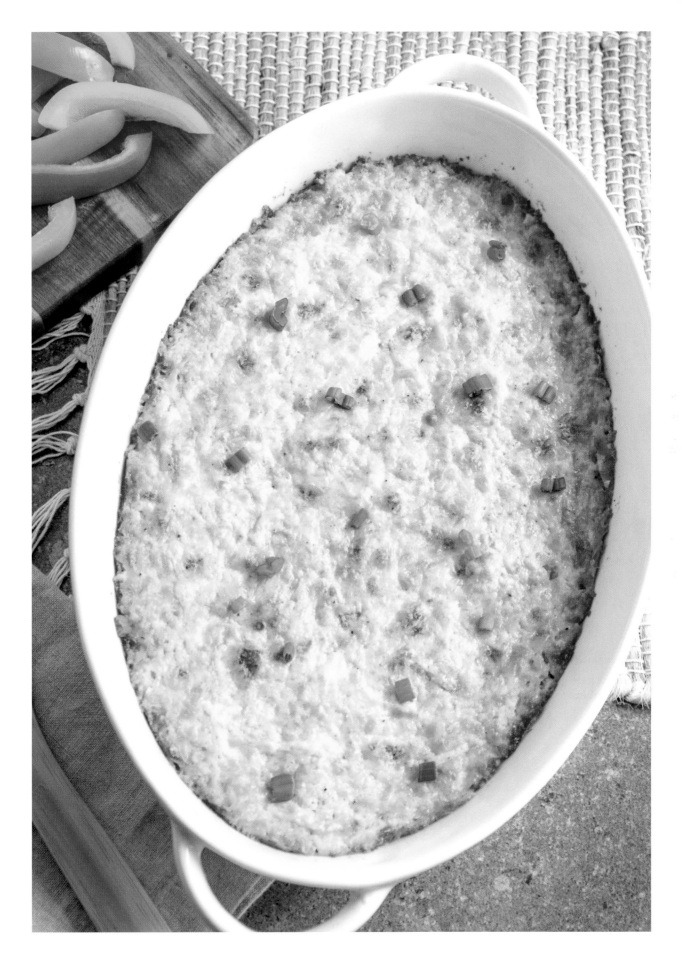

Cheesy Sausage Balls

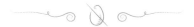

yield: 6 servings

prep time: 10 minutes

cook time: 25 minutes

When I was growing up, sausage balls could always be found on the table during the holidays, alongside finger foods and desserts. Everyone in my family—including myself years later— made sausage balls with Bisquick. This keto version tastes just as good as the original—or maybe even better!

1 pound bulk breakfast sausage

1½ cups shredded sharp cheddar cheese

1 cup finely ground blanched almond flour

1 tablespoon baking powder

1. Preheat the oven to 375°F. Line a sheet pan with parchment paper.

2. Place all the ingredients in a large bowl. Using your hands, mix everything together until well combined but not overmixed.

3. Using a tablespoon or small cookie scoop, form the mixture into 1-inch balls and place on the lined sheet pan. Bake for 20 to 25 minutes, until the sausage balls are crispy around the edges and golden brown on top. Leftovers can be stored in an airtight container in the refrigerator for up to 5 days.

Note:

You can use a stand mixer with a dough hook to make the job of mixing the ingredients easier.

NET CARBS 3.1g				
calories	fat	protein	carbs	fiber
527	45.2g	22.4g	5.7g	2.6g

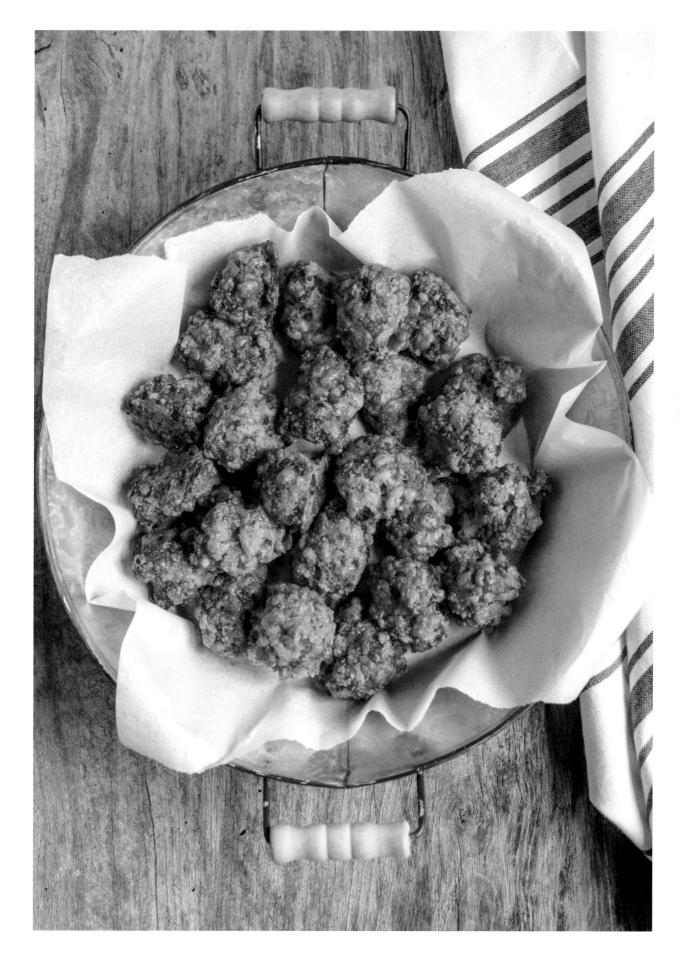

Pimento Cheese

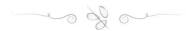

yield: 8 servings

prep time: 20 minutes, plus 1 hour to chill

If you live in the South, you know that prepared pimento cheese is readily available in stores, but it doesn't begin to compare with the goodness of homemade. The best pimento cheese is made with freshly shredded cheese. Don't skip that step; it really makes a difference!

1 (8-ounce) block sharp cheddar cheese

1 (8-ounce) block mild cheddar cheese

1 cup mayonnaise

1 (4-ounce) jar diced pimentos, drained

3 ounces cream cheese (6 tablespoons), softened

1 tablespoon finely chopped onions

1 tablespoon dill relish

½ teaspoon onion powder

¼ teaspoon garlic powder

¼ teaspoon ground black pepper

SERVING SUGGESTIONS:

Sliced bell peppers or celery

Pork rinds

1. Using the large holes on the side of a box grater, shred the cheeses into a large bowl.

2. Add the rest of the ingredients to the bowl with the shredded cheese and mix with a spoon until well combined. Refrigerate for at least 1 hour before serving. Leftovers can be stored in an airtight container in the refrigerator for up to a week.

NET CARBS 2.9g				
calories	fat	protein	carbs	fiber
464	45.5g	14g	3.3g	0.4g

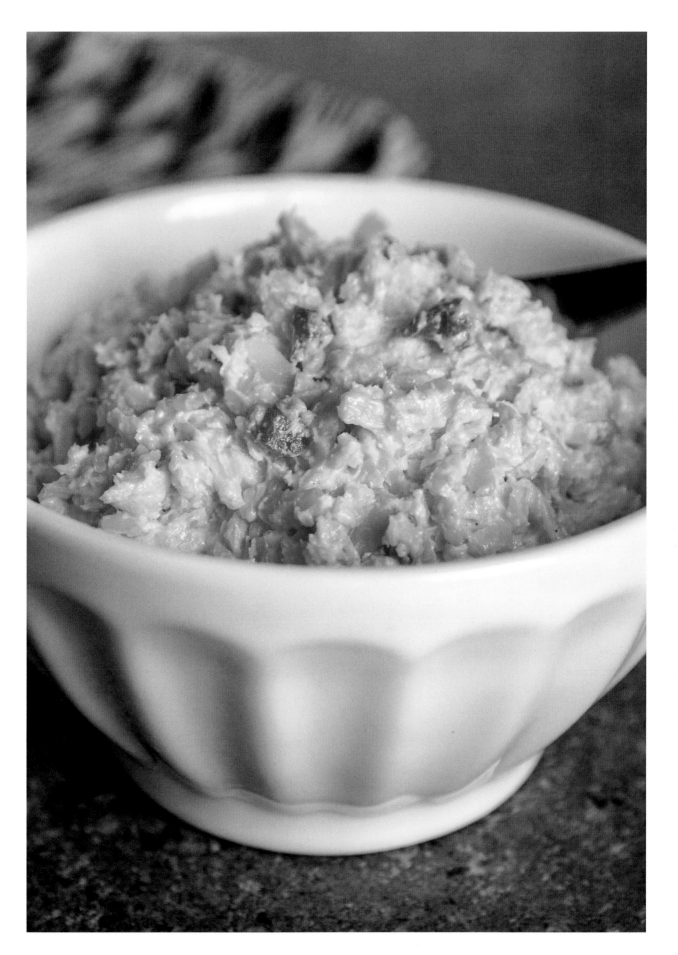

Dill Pickle Chips

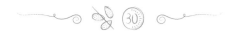

yield: 4 servings

prep time: 10 minutes

cook time: 20 minutes

This recipe combines two Southern favorites: pickles and fried foods. There was a restaurant called Toots in my college town, Bowling Green, Kentucky, that had the best fried dill pickle chips in the world! When my husband and I were dating, we went there every time he came to town—it became our place. When I made this version, he gave it the thumbs-up! We like dipping these chips in ranch dressing.

High-quality oil, for frying

1 large egg

2 tablespoons heavy whipping cream

1 cup finely crushed pork rinds

½ cup grated Parmesan cheese

½ teaspoon garlic powder

¼ teaspoon paprika

⅛ teaspoon cayenne pepper

1 (16-ounce) jar dill pickle rounds, drained

1 cup Ranch Dressing (page 274) or other dip of choice, for serving (optional)

SPECIAL EQUIPMENT:

Candy thermometer

1. Attach a candy thermometer to a Dutch oven or other large heavy pot, then pour in 2 inches of oil and set over medium-high heat. Heat the oil to 375°F.

2. In a shallow dish, whisk together the egg and cream. In another shallow dish, use a fork to combine the pork rinds, Parmesan cheese, garlic powder, paprika, and cayenne.

3. In small batches, dip the pickles in the egg wash and then in the pork rind mixture, making sure to press the crumbs onto all sides of the pickles.

4. Working in batches, carefully place the pickles in the hot oil and fry until golden brown, 1 to 2 minutes per side. Use a mesh skimmer or slotted spoon to remove the pickles from the oil and place on a paper towel-lined plate to drain. Serve immediately with the dipping sauce of your choice. The pickle chips are best eaten the day they are made.

NET CARBS 3.9g				
calories	fat	protein	carbs	fiber
172	9.1g	14.1g	5.2g	1.2g

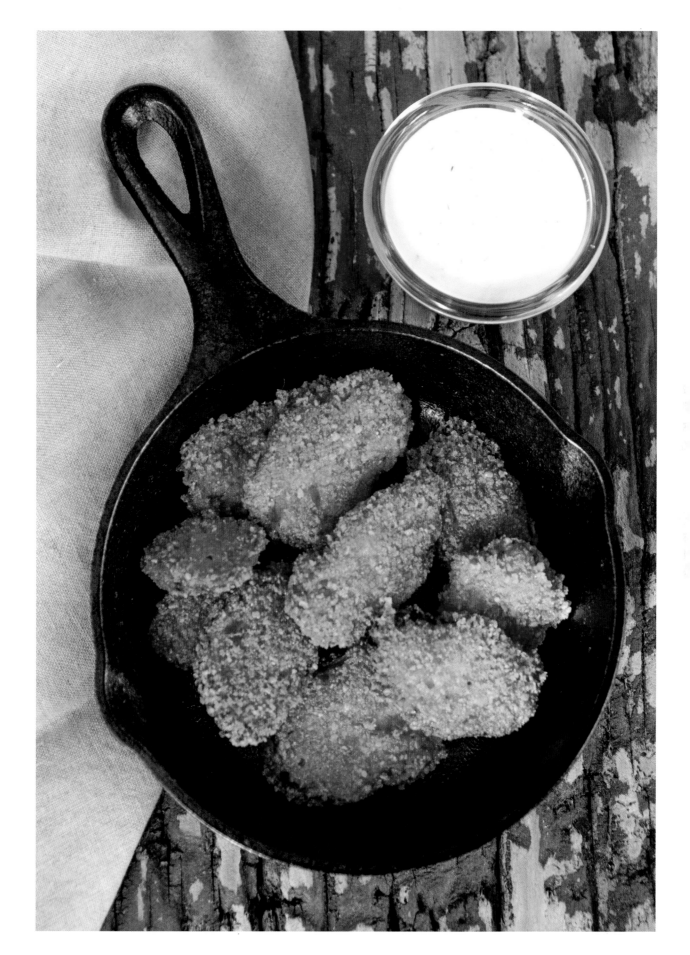

Cheese Crisps

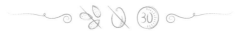

yield: 2 servings

prep time: 5 minutes

cook time: 14 minutes

These lacy cheese crisps are great when you're craving something crunchy. There are so many uses for them—on a taco salad, with a dip, or just as a snack. You can season them however you like. I like to use Italian seasoning or leave them plain.

1 cup shredded sharp cheddar cheese

1 tablespoon seasoning(s) of choice (optional)

1. Preheat the oven to 375°F. Line a sheet pan with parchment paper.

2. Drop tablespoons of the cheese onto the lined sheet pan, spacing them at least 2 inches apart. Sprinkle with the seasoning of your choice, if desired.

3. Bake for 12 to 14 minutes, until the crisps are golden brown and the desired crispness; watch closely at the end of the baking time to avoid burning them. Allow to cool before removing from the parchment paper; they will get crispier as they cool. The crisps are best if eaten the day they are made.

Note:

You also can make these crisps in the microwave. Line a microwave-safe plate with parchment paper. Spoon small piles of cheese onto the parchment, spacing them 2 inches apart. Microwave for 1 minute 30 seconds or until the crisps start to brown. Allow to cool before removing from the parchment paper.

NET CARBS 1.7g				
calories	fat	protein	carbs	fiber
228	18.8g	12.9g	1.7g	0g

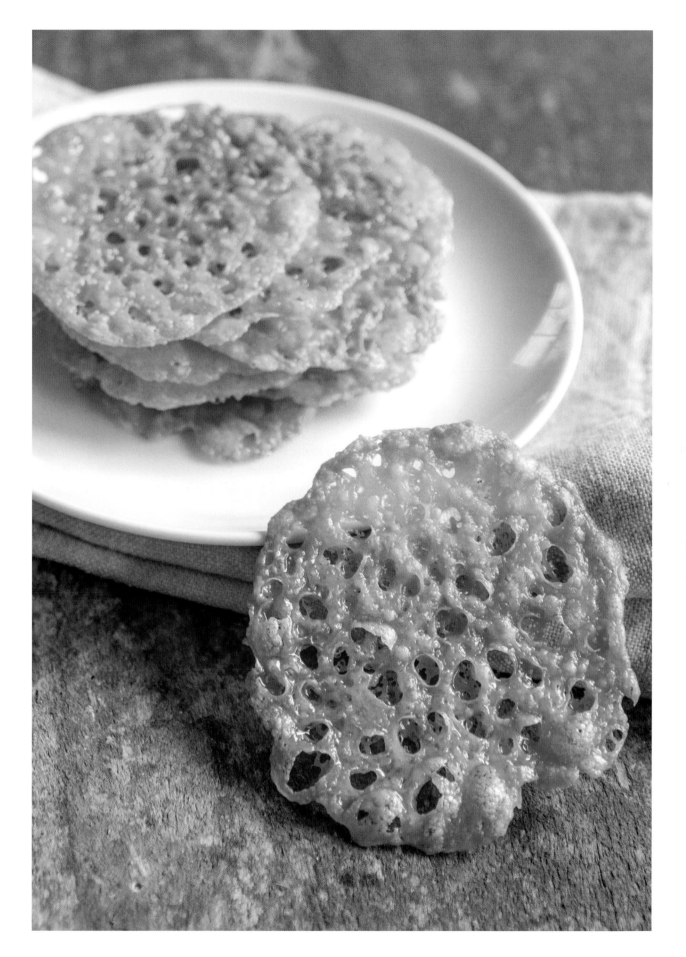

Sweet Pepper Poppers

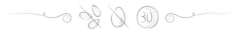

yield: 4 servings

prep time: 10 minutes

cook time: 20 minutes

Southerners enjoy entertaining, and that often involves serving lots of hot dips and finger foods. During football season, you frequently can find jalapeño poppers on the appetizer table. My family likes jalapeño poppers, but sometimes we want something a little different. These sweet pepper poppers are so yummy! They're also great for people who don't like the heat of jalapeños.

12 mini sweet peppers

1 (8-ounce) package cream cheese, softened

5 slices bacon, cooked and crumbled

1 green onion, thinly sliced

¼ teaspoon ground black pepper

1. Preheat the oven to 400°F. Line a sheet pan with parchment paper.

2. Cut each sweet pepper in half lengthwise, then remove and discard the seeds; set the peppers aside.

3. In a small bowl, mix together the cream cheese, bacon, green onion (reserve some of the slices for garnish, if desired), and black pepper. Spoon the mixture into the sweet pepper halves.

4. Place the stuffed peppers on the lined sheet pan and bake for 20 minutes, until the peppers are tender and the tops are starting to brown. Garnish with the reserved green onion slices, if desired.

NET CARBS 4.4g				
calories	fat	protein	carbs	fiber
163	11.9g	6.5g	5.4g	1g

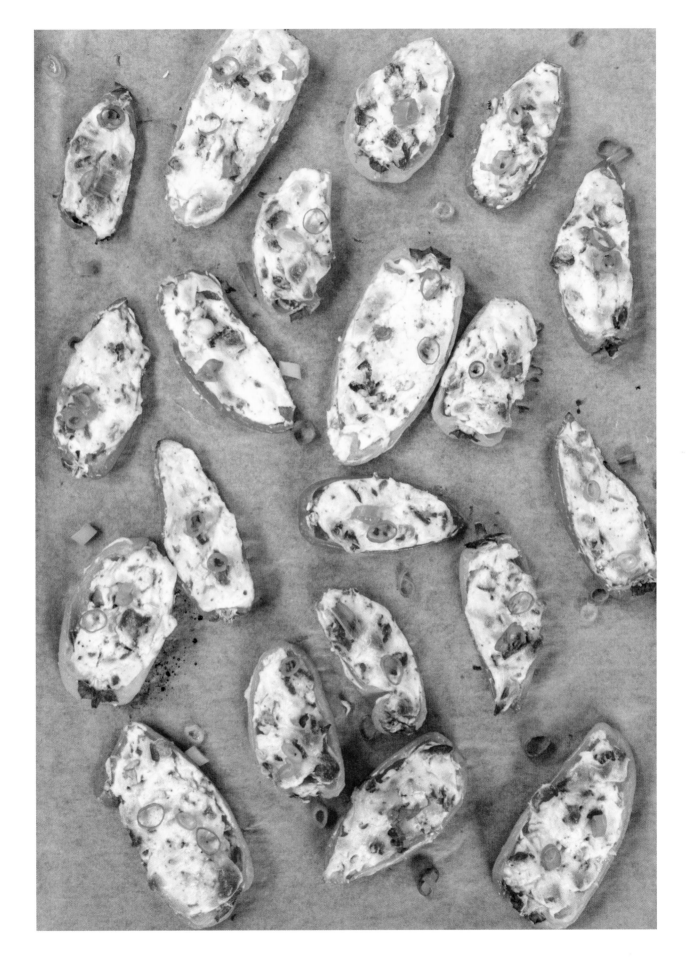

Hushpuppies

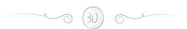

*yield: 10 hushpuppies
(2 per serving)*

prep time: 10 minutes

cook time: 15 minutes

High-quality oil, for frying

1 cup finely ground blanched almond flour

1 tablespoon coconut flour

1 teaspoon baking powder

½ teaspoon salt

¼ cup finely chopped onions

¼ cup heavy whipping cream

1 large egg, beaten

SPECIAL EQUIPMENT:
Candy thermometer

Yes, you read that right. This is a recipe for hushpuppies, and they taste like the real deal! When I developed this recipe, I was so excited about how close they are to the restaurant hushpuppies I ate growing up. For the best texture, you'll want to eat these the same day you make them.

1. Attach a candy thermometer to a Dutch oven or other large heavy pot, then pour in 3 inches of oil and set over medium-high heat. Heat the oil to 375°F.

2. In a medium-sized bowl, stir together the almond flour, coconut flour, baking powder, and salt. Stir in the rest of the ingredients and mix until blended. Do not overmix.

3. Use a tablespoon-sized cookie scoop to gently drop the batter into the hot oil. Don't overcrowd the hushpuppies; cook them in two batches. Fry for 3 minutes, then use a mesh skimmer or slotted spoon to turn and fry them for 3 more minutes or until golden brown on all sides.

4. Use the skimmer or slotted spoon to remove the hushpuppies from the oil and place on a paper towel–lined plate to drain. They are best served immediately.

NET CARBS 2.5g				
calories	fat	protein	carbs	fiber
172	14g	6g	5.1g	2.6g

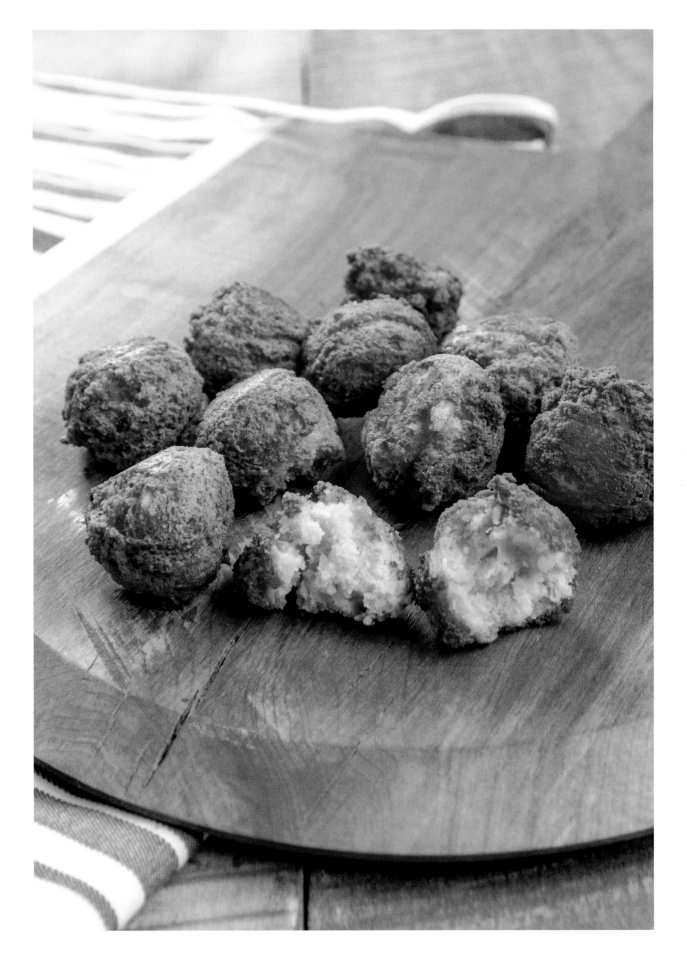

Deviled Eggs

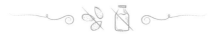

yield: 12 egg halves
(3 per serving)

prep time: 20 minutes

cook time: 15 minutes

Although this seems like a simple recipe, deviled eggs are special to me. When I was young, I would sit with my grandma at the kitchen table and watch her make the perfect deviled eggs. She didn't use any fancy equipment, and her eggs always peeled effortlessly. I would watch her patiently mash the yolks with a fork until the filling was perfectly smooth. I have nothing against food processors—I love kitchen appliances—but when it comes to deviled eggs, I'm always going to make them like Grandma did.

6 large eggs

¼ cup mayonnaise

1 tablespoon dill relish

1 teaspoon prepared yellow mustard

Salt and ground black pepper

Paprika, for garnish (optional)

1. Place the eggs in a single layer in a medium-sized saucepan. Cover with water by 3 inches. Bring to a boil over high heat. Cover the pan and remove from the heat; let the eggs sit in the hot water for 15 minutes.

2. Rinse the eggs with cold water until cool. Crack the shells and gently peel the eggs under cold running water. Slice the eggs in half lengthwise and carefully remove the yolks.

3. Put the yolks in a small bowl and use a fork to mash them with the mayonnaise, relish, and mustard until the filling is smooth. Season to taste with salt and pepper.

4. Spoon the yolk mixture into the egg white halves and sprinkle with paprika, if desired. Refrigerate until ready to serve. The eggs can be stored in an airtight container in the refrigerator for up to 3 days.

Note:
If you like your deviled eggs with a touch of sweetness, you can add a few drops of liquid sweetener, such as stevia, to the yolk mixture in Step 3.

NET CARBS 0.6g				
calories	fat	protein	carbs	fiber
209	18.3g	9.5g	0.6g	0.1g

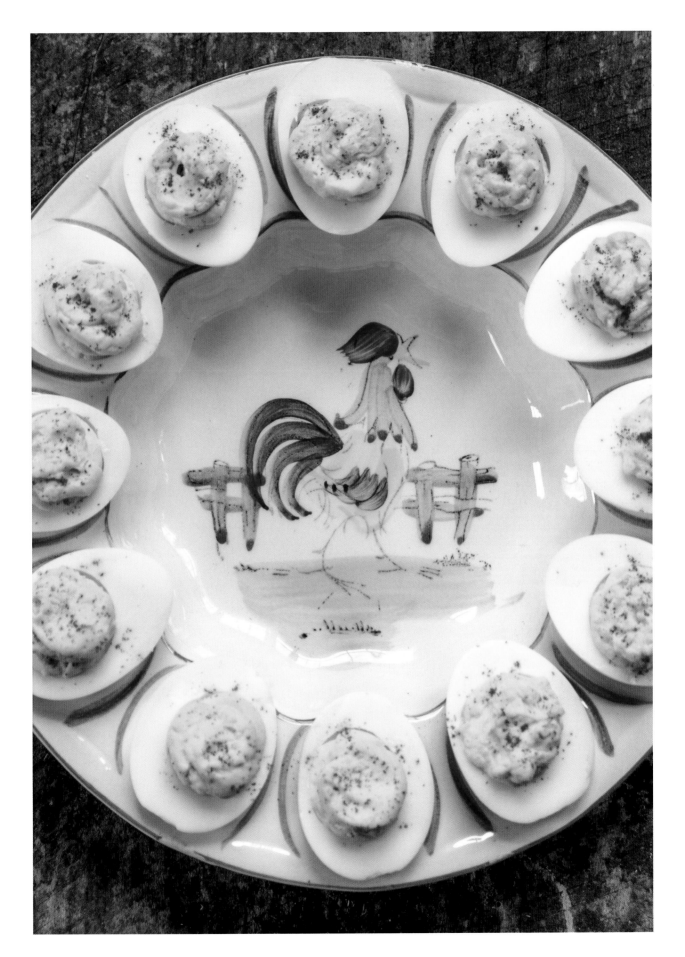

Pecan Ranch Cheese Ball

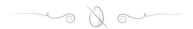

yield: 8 servings

prep time: 15 minutes, plus time to chill overnight

2 (8-ounce) packages cream cheese, softened

1 cup shredded sharp cheddar cheese

2 tablespoons Ranch Seasoning (page 273)

1 cup chopped raw pecans

SERVING SUGGESTIONS:

Celery sticks

Mini sweet peppers

Pork rinds

This is a family favorite that I serve during the holidays and at parties. It's always a big hit. No respectable cheese ball in the South would be coated with anything other than pecans.

1. Put the cream cheese, cheddar cheese, and ranch seasoning in a medium-sized bowl. Using a spoon, mix the ingredients together until well blended.

2. Shape the mixture into a ball or disc shape and roll it in the pecans. Wrap and refrigerate overnight before serving.

3. Serve with the scoopers of your choice. Leftovers can be stored in an airtight container in the refrigerator for up to 5 days.

NET CARBS 5.1g				
calories	fat	protein	carbs	fiber
303	26.8g	9.1g	10.8g	1.8g

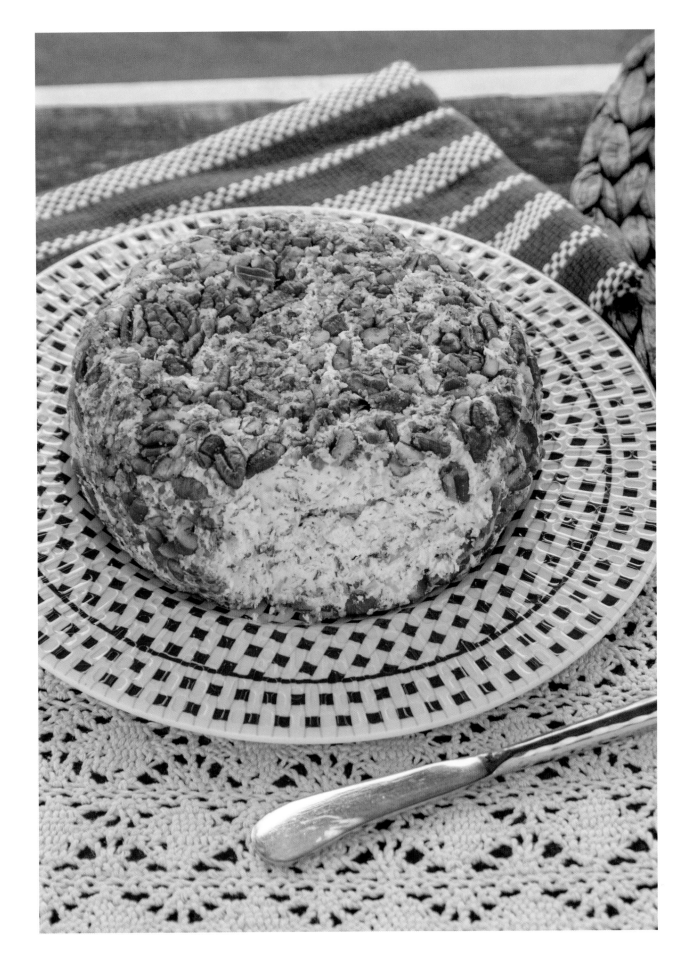

Pulled Pork Buffalo Dip for Two

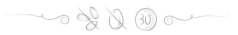

yield: 2 servings

prep time: 5 minutes

cook time: 15 minutes

Here's another way to use leftover Slow Cooker Pulled Pork. Dips are the ultimate Southern party food—or at least I think so. Sometimes you've got to have some Buffalo dip, but there isn't a party to take it to. Here's your answer: Pulled Pork Buffalo Dip for Two! And it's a breeze to whip up. It's great served with celery sticks and/or pork rinds.

1 cup Slow Cooker Pulled Pork (page 158)

4 ounces cream cheese (½ cup), softened

¼ cup Buffalo Sauce (page 275)

½ cup shredded cheddar cheese

1. Preheat the oven to 375°F.

2. In a small bowl, mix together the pulled pork, cream cheese, and Buffalo sauce. Spread the mixture in a small baking dish (with a capacity of about 2 cups), then top with the cheddar cheese.

3. Bake for 15 minutes, until the top is browned and the edges are bubbling. Serve with the dippers of your choice.

SERVING SUGGESTIONS:

Celery sticks

Pork rinds

Note:

Shredded chicken may be substituted for the pulled pork.

NET CARBS 1.9g				
calories	fat	protein	carbs	fiber
377	32.3g	16.7g	2g	0g

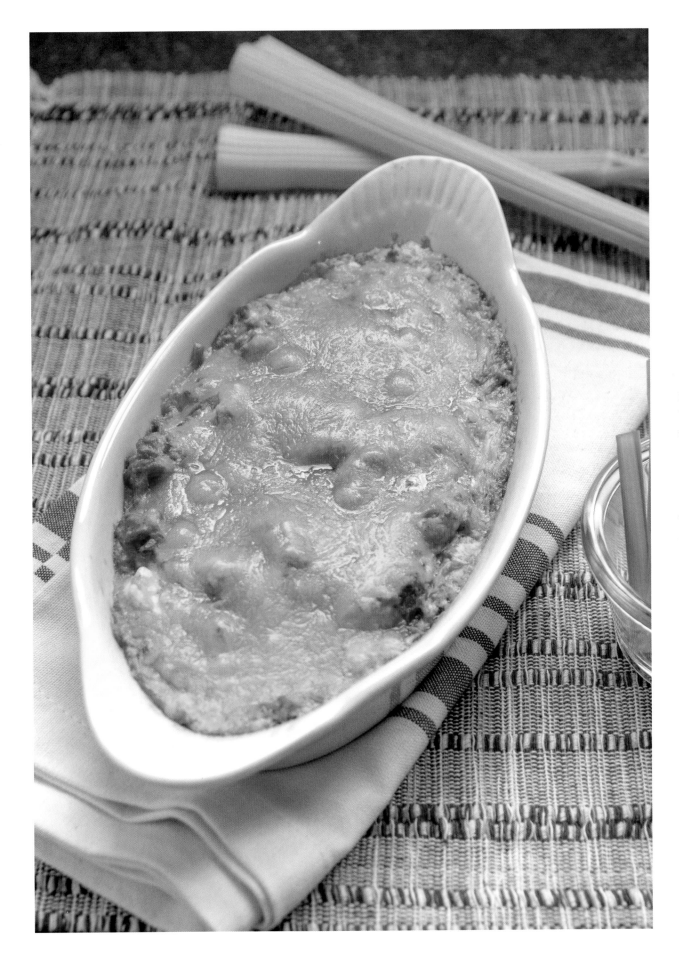

Cucumber Finger Sandwiches

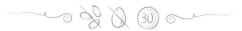

yield: 4 servings

prep time: 10 minutes

The reason I included such an easy recipe is to get you thinking about using vegetables such as cucumbers as a replacement for bread or crackers. After all, the filling is what makes a great sandwich! These little finger sandwiches make a nice lunch or tray of appetizers. Use your imagination and try filling them with a variety of meats and cheeses.

1 medium English cucumber

2 ounces cream cheese (¼ cup), softened

2 to 3 slices sharp cheddar cheese, cut into 1-inch pieces

4 slices bacon, cooked and cut crosswise into 1-inch pieces

Slice the cucumber crosswise into rounds about ¼ inch thick. Spread the cream cheese on half of the cucumber slices, then top each with a piece of cheese and a piece of bacon. Place the remainder of the cucumber slices on top to make sandwiches. Serve immediately or cover and refrigerate before serving. These sandwiches should be eaten the day they are made or they will become soggy.

Note:

You can use mayonnaise in place of the cream cheese, if desired.

NET CARBS 3.1g				
calories	fat	protein	carbs	fiber
187	14.7g	10.1g	3.4g	0.4g

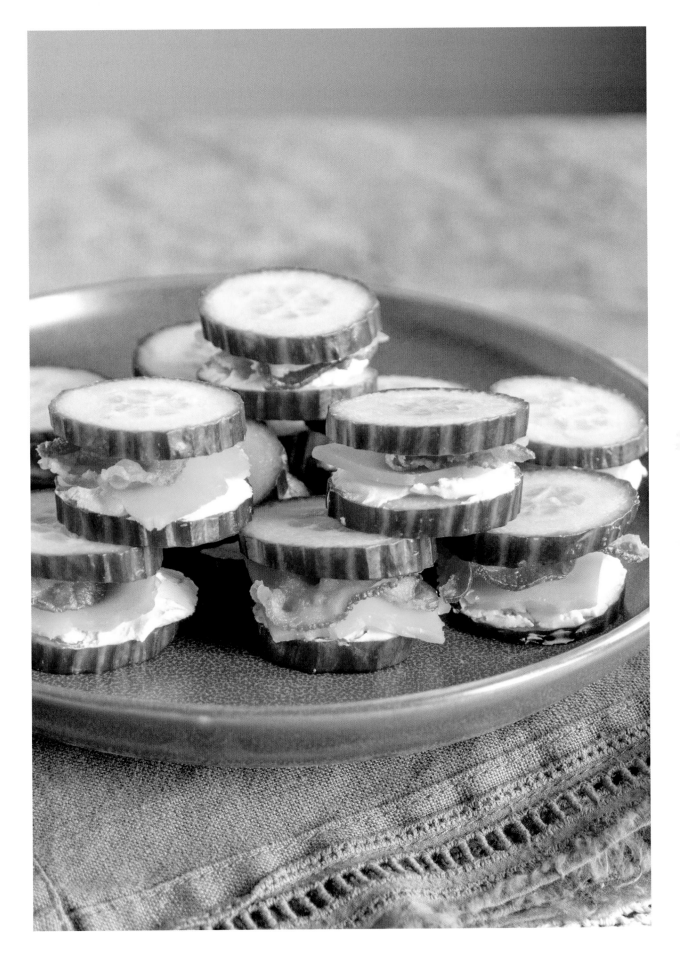

Baked BLT Dip

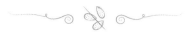

yield: 8 servings

prep time: 20 minutes

cook time: 25 minutes

Southerners love hot dips...so, yes, it's another dip recipe! I mean, can you really have too many hot dips? This BLT Dip is sure to be a hit because you can't go wrong with any dip that has bacon in it!

1 (8-ounce) package cream cheese, softened

½ cup mayonnaise

½ cup sour cream

10 slices bacon, cooked and cut into small pieces

1 medium tomato, seeded and finely diced

¼ cup sliced green onions

1 cup shredded cheddar cheese

FOR GARNISH:

Shredded lettuce

Diced tomatoes

Bacon pieces

Sliced green onions

SERVING SUGGESTIONS:

Celery sticks

Mini sweet peppers

Pork rinds

1. Preheat the oven to 350°F. Grease a 9-inch round baking dish with oil.

2. In a medium-sized bowl, stir together the cream cheese, mayonnaise, and sour cream until thoroughly combined. Add the bacon, tomato, green onions, and cheddar cheese and stir until well combined.

3. Spread the mixture evenly in the prepared baking dish. Bake for 20 to 25 minutes, until the dip is lightly browned on top and bubbling around the edges.

4. Garnish with shredded lettuce, diced tomatoes, bacon pieces, and sliced green onions. Serve with the dippers of your choice. Leftovers can be stored in an airtight container in the refrigerator for up to 5 days.

NET CARBS 2g				
calories	fat	protein	carbs	fiber
329	29.9g	10.3g	2.2g	0.3g

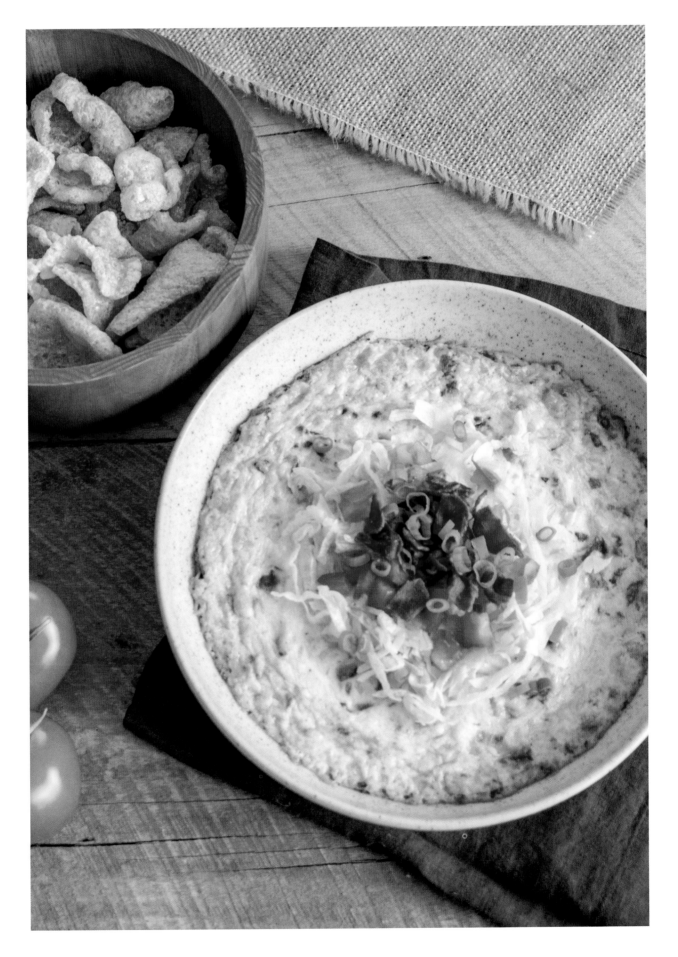

Bacon-Stuffed Mushrooms

*yield: 16 stuffed mushrooms
(4 per serving)*
prep time: 20 minutes
cook time: 40 minutes

Stuffed mushrooms always tempt me when I see them on restaurant menus, but some of them contain hidden carbs, such as breadcrumbs. I like making my own stuffed mushrooms because I know exactly what goes into them. I've found that breadcrumbs aren't even necessary; these mushrooms are delicious without them. They are great served on their own and also are wonderful paired with steak!

16 large white mushrooms (1½ to 2 inches in diameter)

1 tablespoon avocado oil

8 slices bacon, diced

¼ cup finely chopped green onions

1 clove garlic, minced

1 (8-ounce) package cream cheese, cubed

Sliced green onions, for garnish (optional)

1. Preheat the oven to 350°F. Line a sheet pan with parchment paper.

2. Clean the mushrooms and pat them dry. Remove the stems and chop them; set aside. Set the mushroom caps on the lined sheet pan, stem side up.

3. Heat the oil in a medium-sized skillet over medium heat. Add the bacon, chopped mushroom stems, green onions, and garlic and cook until the bacon is crispy and the mushroom stems are tender. Reduce the heat to low.

4. Add the cream cheese to the skillet and stir until melted and well incorporated into the other ingredients. Remove the skillet from the heat.

5. Fill each mushroom with a spoonful of the cream cheese mixture and place on the lined sheet pan.

6. Bake the stuffed mushrooms for 30 minutes, or until tender and slightly browned on top. This could take less time depending on how large your mushrooms are. Garnish with sliced green onions before serving, if desired.

NET CARBS 3.6g				
calories	fat	protein	carbs	fiber
305	25g	14g	4.7g	1.1g

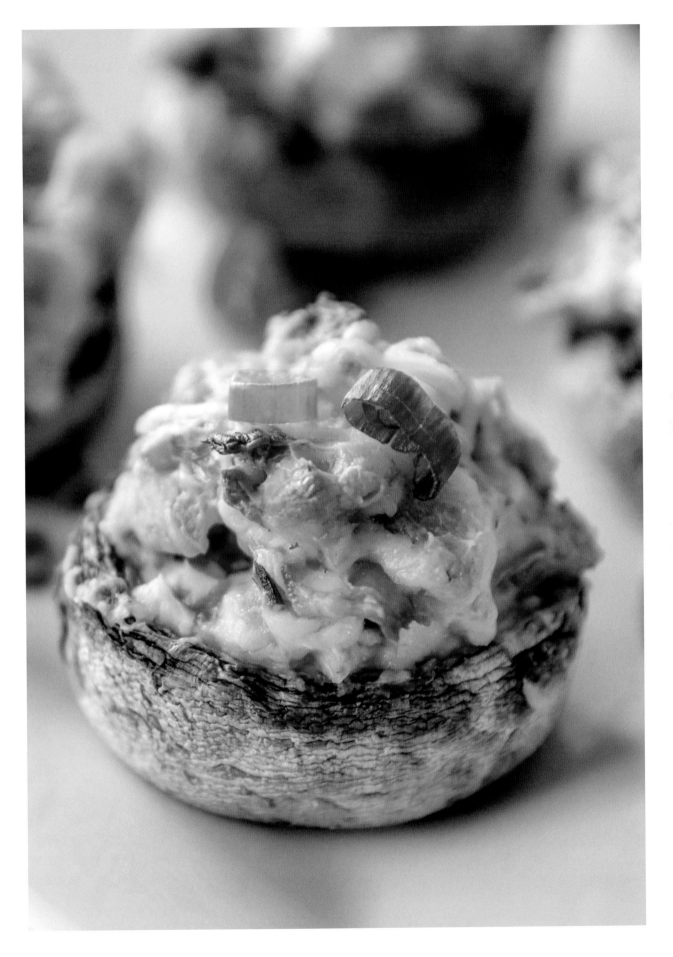

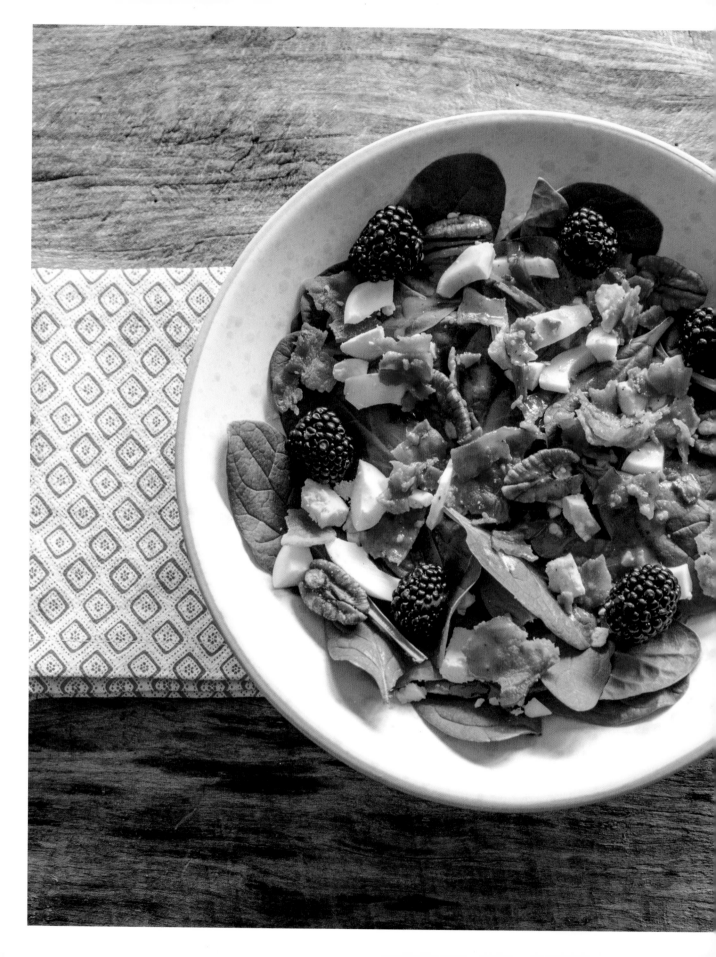

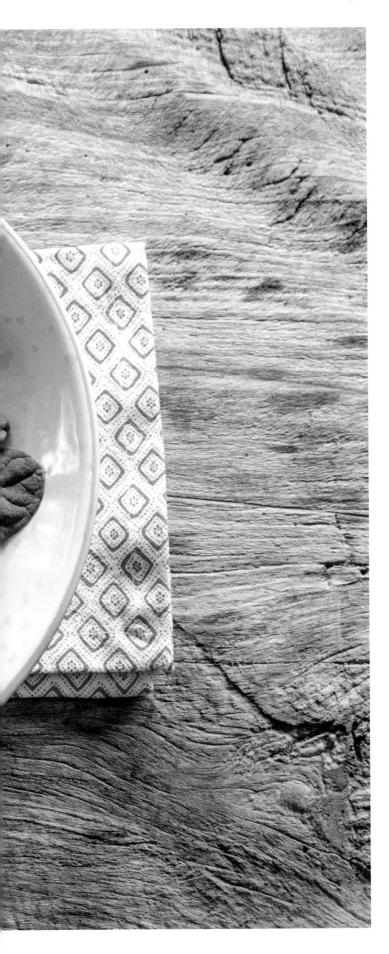

Soups & Salads

Broccoli Cheese Soup

yield: 4 servings

prep time: 5 minutes

cook time: 20 minutes

Soup is a comfort food that we love to eat year-round, and broccoli cheese soup is one of our favorites—it's so quick and easy to make. My husband says he likes this version just as much as the broccoli cheese soup he orders from Ruby Tuesday, a national (and even international) restaurant chain that got its start in Knoxville, near the campus of the University of Tennessee. I like to make a double batch and eat the leftovers for lunch.

3 tablespoons salted butter

½ cup chopped white onions

2 cloves garlic, minced

1 (16-ounce) bag frozen broccoli florets

3 cups vegetable broth

2 cups shredded sharp cheddar cheese, plus extra for garnish

1 cup heavy whipping cream

Salt and ground black pepper

1. Melt the butter in a stockpot over medium heat. Sauté the onions and garlic in the butter until the onions are tender and translucent.

2. Add the broccoli and broth to the pot. Bring to a gentle boil over high heat, then reduce the heat to maintain a simmer and continue cooking until the broccoli is tender, stirring occasionally, about 15 minutes.

3. Turn the heat down to the lowest setting and add the cheese and cream to the pot. Stir until the cheese is melted and well combined with the rest of the soup.

4. Season to taste with salt and pepper. Serve garnished with extra cheese. Leftovers can be stored in an airtight container in the refrigerator for up to 5 days.

NET CARBS 7.7g				
calories	fat	protein	carbs	fiber
577	50.3g	16.5g	10.8g	3.1g

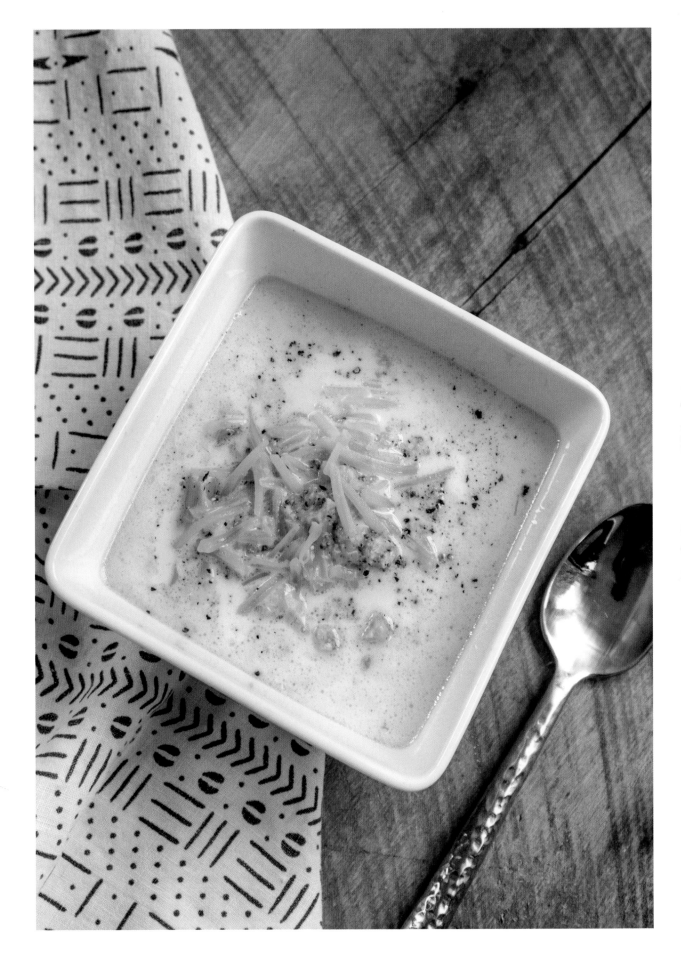

Loaded Fauxtato Soup

yield: 4 servings

prep time: 5 minutes

cook time: 20 minutes

This is my daughter's favorite soup. She was always a huge fan of my loaded potato soup, so this keto version became an instant hit. Not a single person I've served it to has missed the potatoes. It is similar in concept to the Broccoli Cheese Soup on page 114 but is thicker and richer and loaded with bacon. Bonus points for being super easy to make!

3 tablespoons salted butter

½ cup chopped white onions

2 cloves garlic, minced

1 (16-ounce) bag frozen cauliflower florets

2 cups vegetable broth

2 cups shredded sharp cheddar cheese, plus extra for garnish

1 cup heavy whipping cream

Salt and ground black pepper

8 slices bacon, cooked and cut into small pieces, for garnish

1. Melt the butter in a stockpot over medium heat. Sauté the onions and garlic in the butter until the onions are tender and translucent.

2. Add the cauliflower and broth to the pot. Bring to a gentle boil over high heat, then reduce the heat to maintain a simmer and continue cooking until the cauliflower is tender, stirring occasionally, about 15 minutes.

3. Turn the heat down to the lowest setting and add the cheese and cream to the pot. Stir until the cheese is melted and well combined with the rest of the soup.

4. Season to taste with salt and pepper. Serve garnished with extra cheese and bacon pieces. Leftovers can be stored in an airtight container in the refrigerator for up to 5 days.

NET CARBS 6.2g				
calories	fat	protein	carbs	fiber
560	44.6g	30.8g	9.4g	3.2g

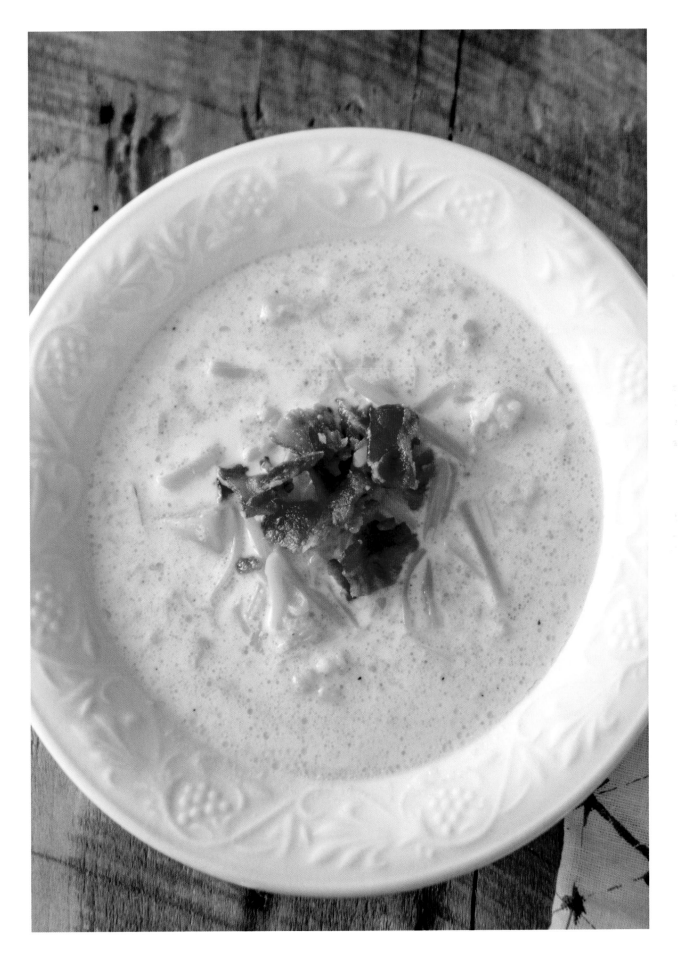

Taco Soup

yield: 8 servings

prep time: 10 minutes

cook time: 1 hour 15 minutes

2 pounds ground beef

½ cup diced onions

2 cloves garlic, minced

1 (8-ounce) package cream cheese, cubed

2 (14½-ounce) cans petite diced tomatoes

1 (15-ounce) can tomato sauce

1 (4-ounce) can diced green chilies

4 cups vegetable broth

2 tablespoons ground cumin

1 tablespoon chili powder

Salt and ground black pepper

FOR GARNISH (optional):

Sour cream

Shredded cheddar cheese

Sliced avocado

Fresh cilantro

For years I made taco soup with corn and pinto beans. Honestly, we don't even miss them in this flavorful alternative! This has been a very popular recipe among the people I've shared it with.

1. Cook the ground beef, onions, and garlic in a stockpot over medium heat, crumbling the meat with a large spoon as it cooks, until the meat is browned, about 10 minutes. Drain the fat, if necessary.

2. Add the cream cheese to the pot. Continue cooking and stirring until the cream cheese is melted and blended with the meat mixture.

3. Stir in the tomatoes, tomato sauce, chilies, broth, cumin, and chili powder. Bring to a boil, then reduce the heat to low and simmer for 1 hour to allow the flavors to come together.

4. Season to taste with salt and pepper. Serve garnished with sour cream, cheddar cheese, avocado slices, and/or cilantro, if desired. Leftovers can be stored in an airtight container in the refrigerator for up to 5 days.

NET CARBS 6.6g				
calories	fat	protein	carbs	fiber
405	29.2g	23.8g	9.1g	2.5g

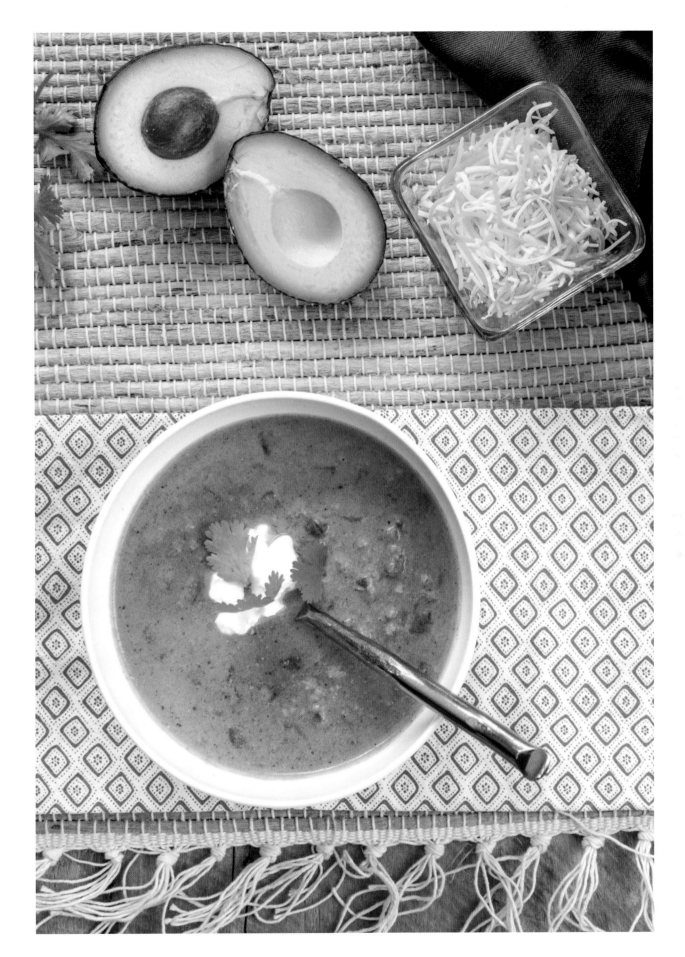

Cheeseburger Soup

yield: 6 servings
prep time: 10 minutes
cook time: 40 minutes

Though this soup doesn't really taste like a cheeseburger, it is hearty and delicious, and it's just as good or even better the next day. It is a keto spin on a cheeseburger soup that I made for years.

2 tablespoons salted butter

½ cup diced celery

¼ cup diced onions

1 clove garlic, minced

1 pound ground beef

3 cups vegetable broth

1 (12-ounce) bag frozen cauliflower florets

1 teaspoon dried basil

1 teaspoon dried parsley

2 cups shredded cheddar cheese

1 cup heavy whipping cream

Salt and ground black pepper

1. Melt the butter in a stockpot over medium heat. Add the celery, onions, and garlic and cook until the celery is tender and the onions are translucent.

2. Add the ground beef to the pot and cook until it is browned, crumbling the meat with a large spoon as it cooks. Drain the fat, if necessary.

3. Add the broth, cauliflower, basil, and parsley to the pot. Bring to a boil, then reduce the heat to maintain a simmer and cook, stirring occasionally, until the cauliflower is tender, about 25 minutes.

4. Turn the heat down to the lowest setting and stir in the cheese and cream. Continue stirring until the cheese is melted.

5. Season to taste with salt and pepper. Leftovers can be stored in an airtight container in the refrigerator for up to 5 days.

NET CARBS 4.4g				
calories	fat	protein	carbs	fiber
544	46.9g	23.8g	6.1g	1.7g

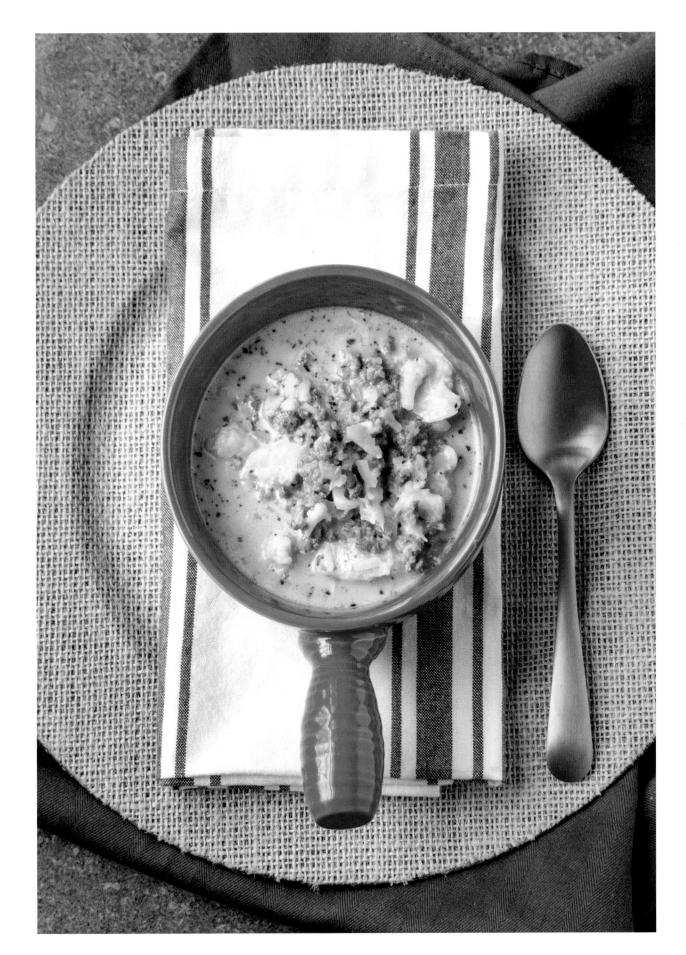

Tomato Basil Soup

yield: 4 servings
prep time: 5 minutes
cook time: 45 minutes

Blessed with a long growing season here in east Tennessee, I have access to fresh basil throughout the summer and into the fall months. What better way to use it than in this comforting dish? This delicious tomato soup is a lot easier to make than you might think!

2 tablespoons salted butter

½ cup chopped onions

2 cloves garlic, minced

1 (28-ounce) can whole peeled tomatoes

1½ cups vegetable broth

¼ cup loosely packed fresh basil leaves, plus extra for garnish if desired

½ cup heavy whipping cream

Salt and ground black pepper

Shredded or grated Parmesan cheese, for garnish (optional)

1. Melt the butter in a stockpot over medium heat. Add the onions and garlic and cook until the onions are tender and translucent.

2. Add the tomatoes, broth, and basil to the pot. Bring to a boil over high heat, then reduce the heat to maintain a simmer and cook for 20 minutes to allow the flavors to come together.

3. Slide the pot off the heat and, using an immersion blender, blend the soup to the desired consistency.

4. Stir in the cream and simmer gently for 15 more minutes before serving.

5. Serve topped with Parmesan cheese and fresh basil leaves, if desired. Leftovers can be stored in an airtight container in the refrigerator for up to 5 days.

Note:

If you don't own an immersion blender, you can use a regular blender or a potato masher instead. If you use a potato masher, you'll end up with a chunkier, rustic-style soup.

NET CARBS 5.9g				
calories	fat	protein	carbs	fiber
205	17.7g	2.9g	10.1g	4.2g

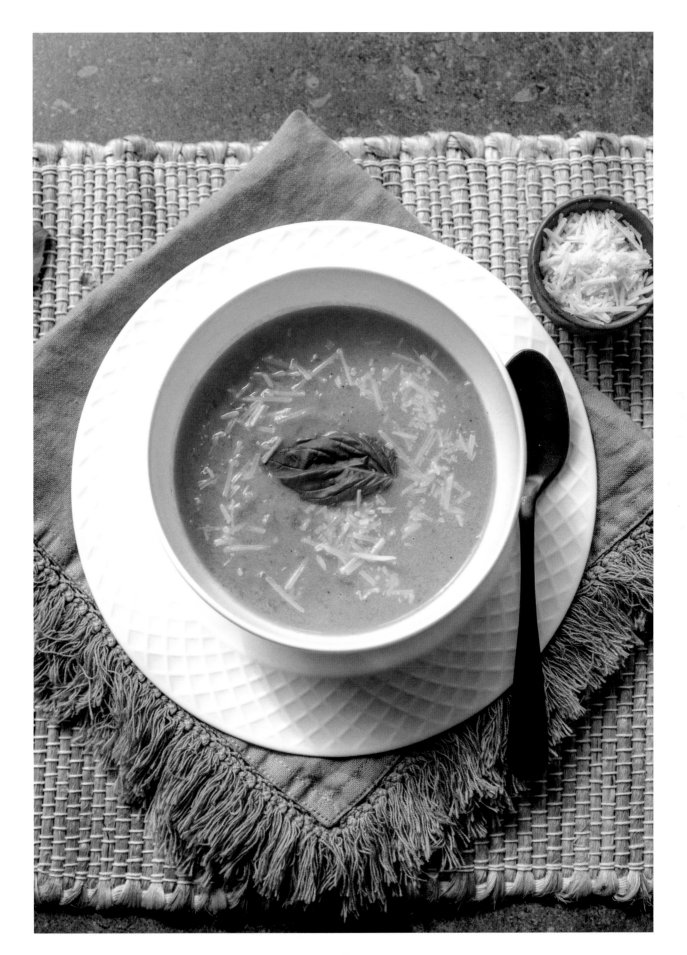

Easy Chili

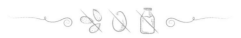

yield: 6 to 8 servings
prep time: 10 minutes
cook time: 35 minutes

When I was growing up, my dad always made the chili at our house. He put spaghetti in his, and although I don't put spaghetti in mine, he still approves of this recipe! This is the same chili I've made for years, minus the beans, and we don't even miss them. Chili doesn't have to be complicated to be good. This chili has great flavor and is easy enough to whip up on a busy weeknight. The leftovers taste even better!

2 pounds ground beef

2 tablespoons dried minced onions

2 teaspoons minced garlic

1 (15-ounce) can tomato sauce

1 (14½-ounce) can petite diced tomatoes

1 cup water

2 tablespoons chili powder

1 tablespoon ground cumin

½ teaspoon salt

½ teaspoon ground black pepper

SUGGESTED TOPPINGS:

Sour cream

Sliced green onions or chopped white onions

Shredded cheddar cheese

1. Cook the ground beef, onions, and garlic in a stockpot over medium heat, crumbling the meat with a large spoon as it cooks, until the meat is browned, about 10 minutes. Drain the fat, if necessary.

2. Add the tomato sauce, tomatoes, water, chili powder, cumin, salt, and pepper to the pot. Bring to a boil, then reduce the heat to low and simmer for 20 minutes to allow the flavors to develop and the chili to thicken slightly.

3. Garnish with the chili topping(s) of your choice and serve. Leftovers can be stored in an airtight container in the refrigerator for up to 5 days.

NET CARBS 6.6g				
calories	fat	protein	carbs	fiber
429	30.8g	27.3g	9g	2.5g
based on 6 servings				

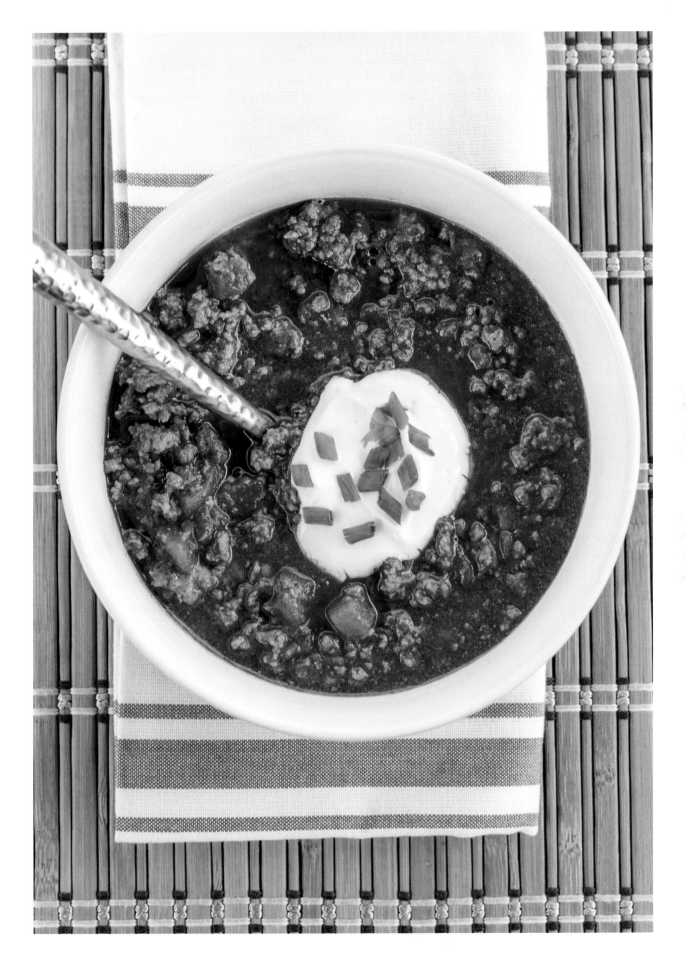

Gumbo

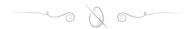

yield: 8 servings

prep time: 20 minutes

cook time: 1 hour 30 minutes

Gumbo is challenging to make keto because it requires a roux, which is traditionally made with wheat flour. I was up for the challenge and created this delicious gumbo with an easy-to-make gluten-free roux. The best part is that the roux doesn't take an hour to prepare!

2 tablespoons avocado oil

1 pound boneless, skinless chicken thighs

Salt and ground black pepper

8 ounces andouille or other smoked sausage, sliced into ½-inch rounds

2 tablespoons salted butter

2 tablespoons finely ground blanched almond flour

1 tablespoon coconut flour

2 cloves garlic, minced

1 medium onion, chopped

1 medium-sized green bell pepper, seeded and chopped

3 ribs celery, diced

6 cups vegetable broth

1 (14½-ounce) can petite diced tomatoes

2 tablespoons Creole Seasoning (page 270)

1 tablespoon dried parsley

2 bay leaves

1½ cups sliced okra

2 recipes Basic Caulirice (page 202), for serving

Sliced green onions, for garnish

Hot sauce, for serving

1. Heat the oil in a stockpot over medium-high heat. Lightly season the chicken with salt and pepper. Cook the chicken and sausage until browned on both sides, then remove the meat, leaving the drippings in the pan. Use a fork to shred the chicken.

2. To make the roux, set the pot with the drippings over medium heat and add the butter, almond flour, and coconut flour. Cook, stirring constantly, until the flour turns dark brown, about 10 minutes.

3. Add the garlic, onion, green pepper, and celery to the pot and cook, stirring occasionally, until the vegetables are tender. Add the shredded chicken and sausage to the pot along with the broth, tomatoes, Creole seasoning, parsley, and bay leaves. Bring to a boil, then lower the heat and simmer for 30 minutes.

4. Add the okra and cook until it is tender and the gumbo is thickened, about 30 more minutes. Season to taste with salt and pepper. Remove the bay leaves.

5. To serve, spoon the gumbo into bowls alongside the caulirice. Garnish with sliced green onions and serve with hot sauce on the side. Leftovers can be stored in an airtight container in the refrigerator for up to 5 days.

Note:

You can add shrimp or crab meat to the gumbo if you like.

NET CARBS 4.2g				
calories	fat	protein	carbs	fiber
523	24.8g	17.7g	6.4g	2.1g

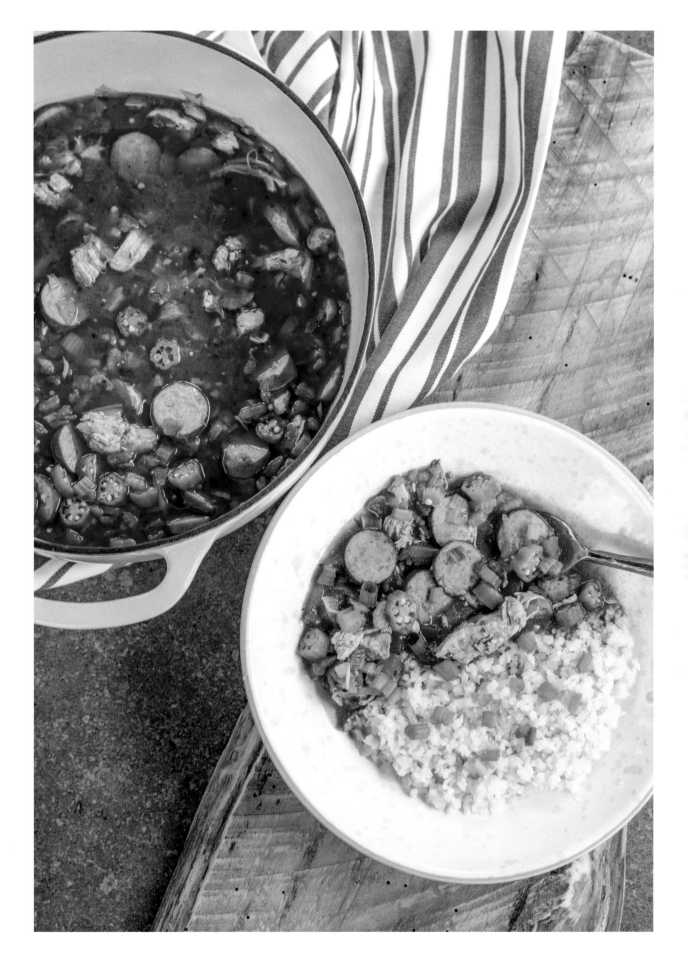

Tuna Salad-Stuffed Peppers

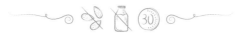

yield: 6 servings

prep time: 20 minutes

Everyone needs a good recipe for tuna salad. It's not fancy, but it's delicious. It makes for the easiest lunches, too.

2 (6-ounce) cans or packages wild-caught tuna (packed in water), drained

2 hard-boiled eggs, peeled and finely diced

1 rib celery, finely diced

1 tablespoon finely chopped onions

½ cup mayonnaise

2 tablespoons dill relish

¼ teaspoon salt

¼ teaspoon ground black pepper

3 red or orange bell peppers, stemmed, cut in half crosswise, and seeded

Fresh dill, for garnish (optional)

1. Place the tuna in a medium-sized bowl and break it up with a fork.

2. To the bowl with the tuna, add the eggs, celery, onions, mayonnaise, relish, salt, and black pepper. Stir until well combined.

3. Spoon the tuna salad into the bell pepper halves. Garnish with dill, if desired. Leftovers can be stored in an airtight container in the refrigerator for up to 2 days.

NET CARBS 3.6g				
calories	fat	protein	carbs	fiber
241	18g	16.6g	5g	1.4g

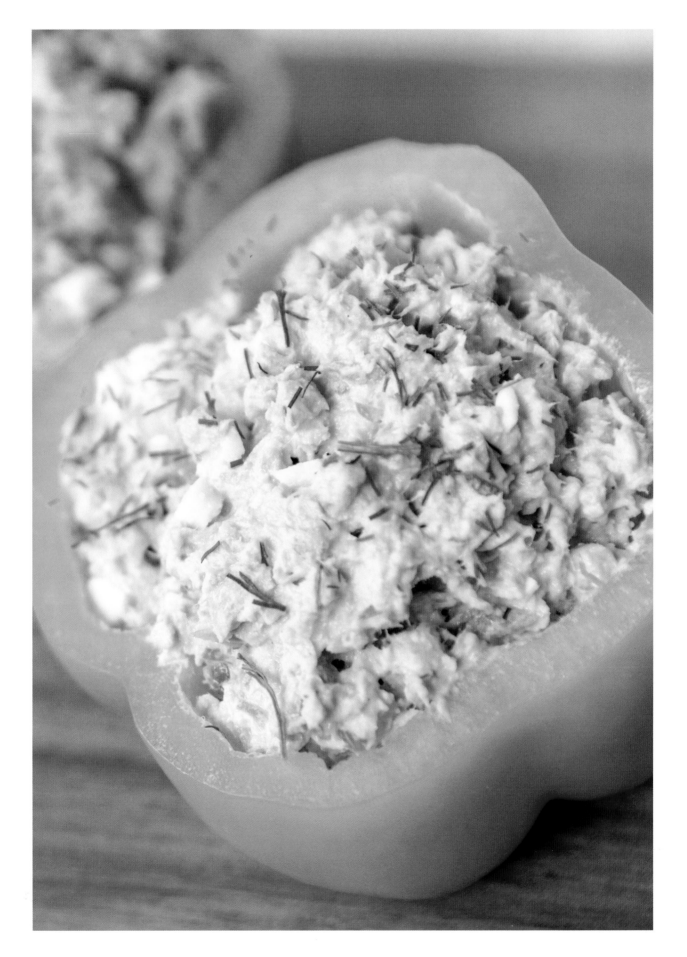

Classic Egg Salad

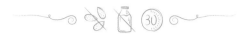

yield: 4 servings
prep time: 10 minutes

When I started keto, I remember thinking, oh my gosh, I can eat egg salad! I was excited because I've always loved egg salad. Of course, I used to eat it on slices of bread. Now I eat it on a bed of spinach or other greens, and it's really satisfying. Sometimes I like a classic egg salad, the way a lot of Southerners prepare it, and sometimes I like an egg salad with a little kick (see the Buffalo variation below). Both versions are good.

6 hard-boiled eggs, peeled and chopped

¼ cup mayonnaise

1 tablespoon finely chopped onions

1 tablespoon dill relish

1 teaspoon prepared yellow mustard

¼ teaspoon paprika

¼ teaspoon ground black pepper

⅛ teaspoon salt

Fresh spinach leaves, for serving (optional)

In a medium-sized mixing bowl, stir together all the ingredients until well incorporated. Serve over spinach leaves, if desired. Leftovers can be stored in an airtight container in the refrigerator for up to 3 days.

Variation:
Buffalo Egg Salad. Stir 2 tablespoons of Buffalo Sauce (page 275) into the Classic Egg Salad. Serve with celery sticks.

NET CARBS 1.1g				
calories	fat	protein	carbs	fiber
213	18.3g	9.6g	1.4g	0.3g

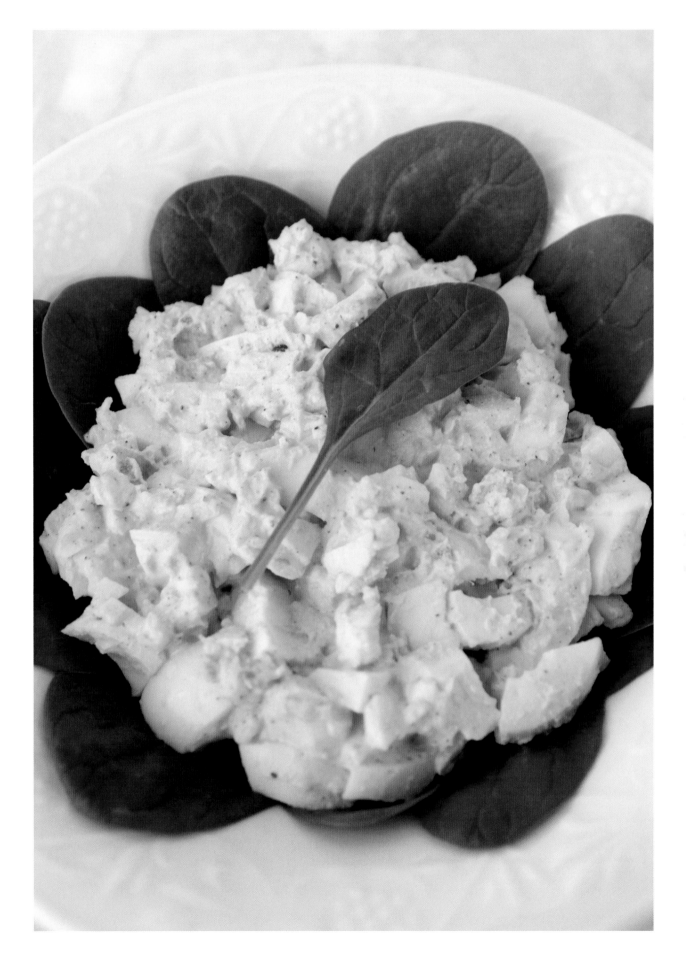

Broccoli Cauliflower Salad

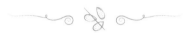

yield: 6 to 8 servings

prep time: 20 minutes, plus 4 hours to chill

Broccoli salad is a classic that has shown up at potlucks for as long as I can remember. Mine is inspired by a broccoli salad recipe that I used to make for summer barbecues. It's almost identical except that I've added cauliflower and replaced the conventional sugar with a keto sweetener. It's just as delicious. Take it to your next get-together; no one will ever know it's keto.

3 cups chopped broccoli florets

3 cups chopped cauliflower florets

½ cup finely diced red onions

1 cup shredded sharp cheddar cheese

½ cup roasted and salted shelled sunflower seeds

10 slices bacon, cooked and crumbled

1 cup mayonnaise

¼ cup granular erythritol

1½ tablespoons apple cider vinegar

1. Put the broccoli, cauliflower, onions, cheese, sunflower seeds, and bacon in a large mixing bowl. Mix until well incorporated.

2. In a small bowl, mix together the mayonnaise, erythritol, and vinegar until well blended. Pour over the broccoli mixture. Toss until well combined.

3. Refrigerate the salad for at least 4 hours or overnight before serving. Leftovers can be stored in an airtight container in the refrigerator for up to 4 days.

NET CARBS 5.3g				
calories	fat	protein	carbs	fiber
277	21.3g	14.6g	8.7g	3.3g
based on 6 servings				

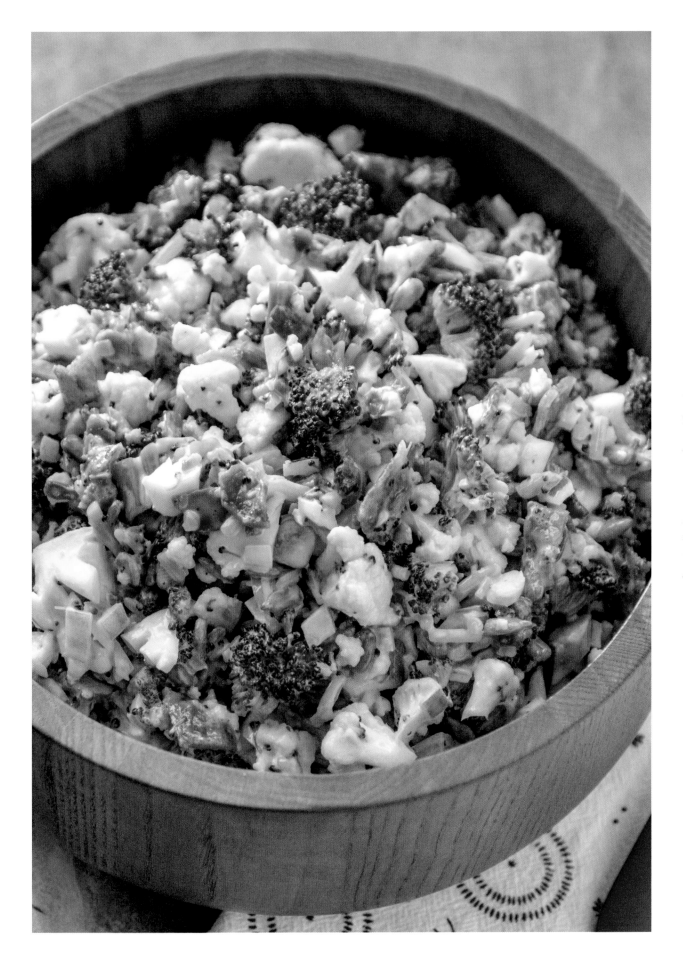

Creamy Coleslaw

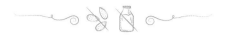

yield: 4 servings

prep time: 5 minutes, plus 2 hours to chill

There's not a whole lot to say about coleslaw, except that I could eat it every day! It's the perfect side dish. It goes with so many things, and it's a breeze to make when you buy a bag of prepped slaw mix. Coleslaw is popular in the South. The taste varies by region. Some coleslaw is sweet, and some is savory. Some is even made with a light vinegar-based dressing rather than the better-known mayonnaise-based version. I grew up enjoying creamy coleslaw with a sweet and tangy flavor; this recipe is very similar. Finely shredded purple cabbage can be added for color.

½ cup mayonnaise

1 tablespoon apple cider vinegar

½ teaspoon salt

½ teaspoon ground black pepper

½ teaspoon garlic powder

1 drop liquid stevia

1 (10-ounce) bag angel hair coleslaw (finely shredded green cabbage)

1. In a medium-sized serving bowl, mix together the mayonnaise, vinegar, salt, pepper, garlic powder, and stevia.

2. Add the shredded cabbage to the mayonnaise mixture. Mix well and refrigerate for at least 2 hours before serving.

3. Serve garnished with freshly ground black pepper. Leftovers can be stored in an airtight container in the refrigerator for up to 5 days.

NET CARBS 2.9g				
calories	fat	protein	carbs	fiber
226	22.3g	0.9g	4.7g	1.8g

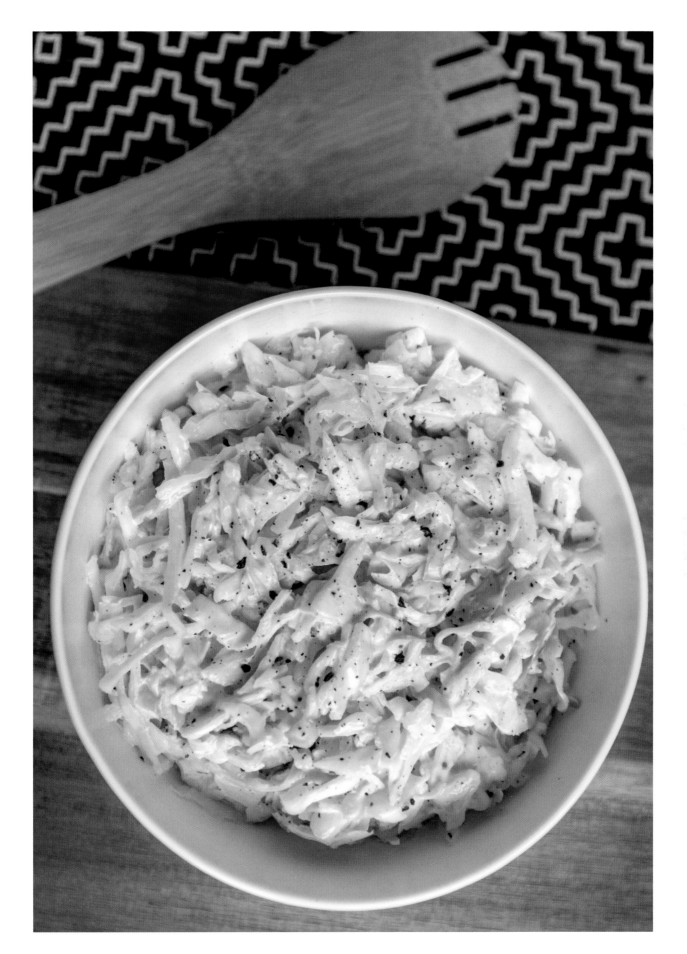

Southern Fauxtato Salad

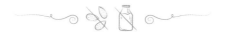

yield: 6 to 8 servings

*prep time: 20 minutes, plus
2 hours to chill*

cook time: 10 minutes

*My mother-in-law makes my favorite potato salad that's made
with real potatoes. It's delicious yet simple. This is my take
on her salad, made with cauliflower. We don't even miss the
potatoes in this recipe!*

2 (10-ounce) bags frozen
cauliflower florets

3 hard-boiled eggs, peeled
and chopped

¼ cup chopped onions

1 rib celery, chopped

1 cup mayonnaise

½ cup dill relish

1 tablespoon prepared yellow
mustard

1 drop liquid stevia

Salt and ground black pepper

1. Cook the cauliflower according to the package directions.
   Drain the excess water and set aside to cool.

2. In a large mixing bowl, mix together the eggs, onions,
   celery, mayonnaise, relish, mustard, and stevia. Stir in
   the cauliflower until well combined. Season to taste with
   salt and pepper.

3. Refrigerate the salad for at least 2 hours before serving.
   Leftovers can be stored in an airtight container in the
   refrigerator for up to 5 days.

NET CARBS 3g				
calories	fat	protein	carbs	fiber
333	35.1g	5.2g	5.5g	2.5g
based on 6 servings				

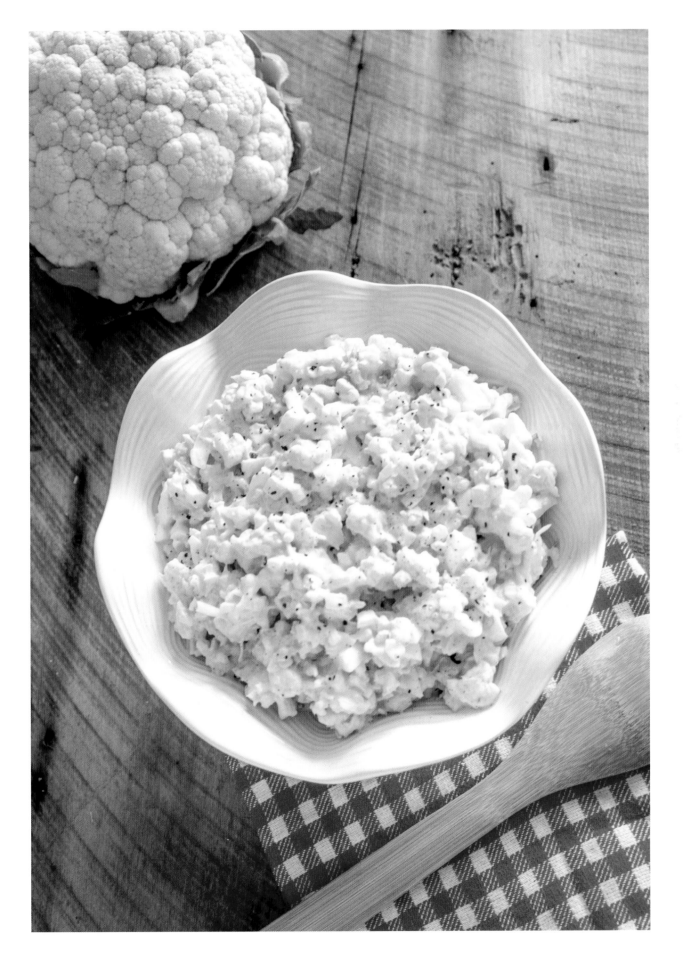

BLT Wedge Salad

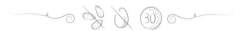

yield: *4 servings*

prep time: *10 minutes*

You can find a classic wedge salad on just about every restaurant menu in the South. But why not make it at home? It really doesn't get any easier than this. If you're a fan of restaurant wedge salads, you'll love this version. And did I mention that it has cheddar cheese on it? Cheese makes everything better!

1 medium head iceberg lettuce

1 cup Ranch Dressing (page 274)

1 cup shredded cheddar cheese

6 slices bacon, cooked and cut into small pieces

8 grape tomatoes, halved

1. Cut the head of lettuce lengthwise into quarters, from core to top, so you have 4 wedges.

2. Place the wedges on a serving platter and drizzle with the dressing. Sprinkle each wedge with one-quarter of the cheese, bacon, and tomatoes and serve.

NET CARBS 6.4g				
calories	fat	protein	carbs	fiber
275	20.4g	14.8g	10g	3.6g

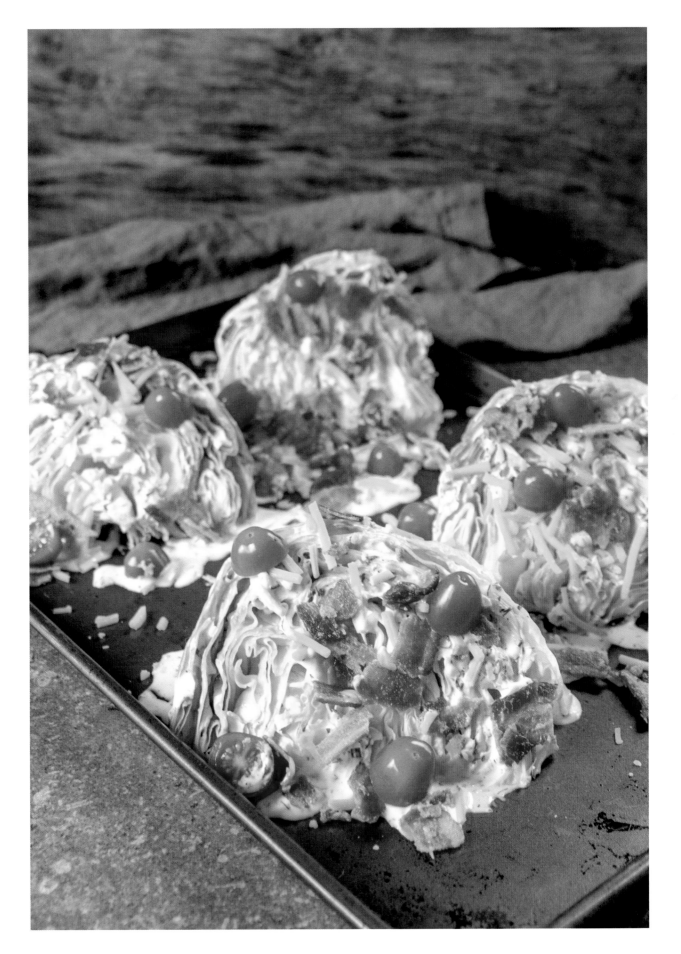

Marinated Cucumber Salad

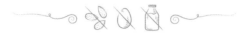

yield: 4 servings

prep time: 10 minutes, plus 2 hours to chill

1 large English cucumber

Salt

½ red onion

½ cup apple cider vinegar

2 tablespoons avocado oil

2 tablespoons granular erythritol

½ teaspoon dried ground oregano

Ground black pepper

Here's another easy salad! Cucumber salad is a refreshing side dish, and it is good packed in lunches.

1. Slice the cucumber crosswise into thin rounds. Place the cucumber slices in a colander over the sink. Sprinkle with salt and allow to sit for 10 minutes. This will cause the excess moisture to drain from the cucumbers.

2. Thinly slice the onion and place in a medium-sized bowl.

3. Use a paper towel to remove any remaining moisture from the cucumber slices, then add the cucumbers to the bowl with the onion slices. Add the vinegar, oil, erythritol, and oregano and gently stir with a spoon. Season to taste with salt and pepper.

4. Place the salad in the refrigerator to chill for at least 2 hours before serving. Leftovers can be stored in an airtight container in the refrigerator for up to 3 days.

NET CARBS 3.5g				
calories	fat	protein	carbs	fiber
85	7.1g	0.7g	4.1g	0.6g

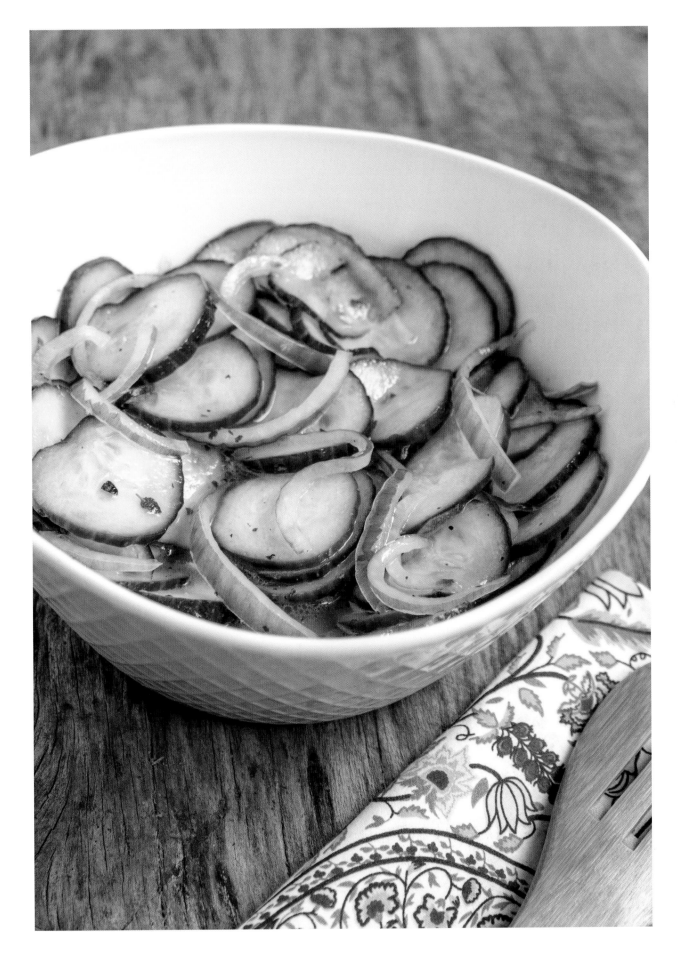

Easy Chicken Salad

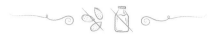

yield: 4 servings

prep time: 10 minutes, plus 1 hour to chill

Chicken salad is so versatile. It's fancy enough to serve at parties yet simple enough for weekday lunches. You'll like the ease of preparation with this one because it uses store-bought rotisserie chicken. I actually think rotisserie chicken makes a better-tasting chicken salad, so it's a win-win.

3 cups shredded rotisserie chicken (see Note)

1 rib celery, finely chopped

¼ cup diced onions

½ cup mayonnaise

2 tablespoons dill relish

Salt and ground black pepper

Lettuce leaves or baby spinach, for serving (optional)

1. Place the chicken, celery, onions, mayonnaise, and relish in a large mixing bowl. Stir well to combine. Season to taste with salt and pepper.

2. Serve on lettuce leaves or a bed of spinach. Leftovers can be stored in an airtight container in the refrigerator for up to 5 days.

Note:

You can use your own cooked and shredded chicken breast and/or thigh meat instead of store-bought rotisserie chicken. However, your salad will not have as much flavor as salad made with rotisserie chicken.

NET CARBS 2.8g				
calories	fat	protein	carbs	fiber
448	29.3g	44.2g	3.1g	0.3g

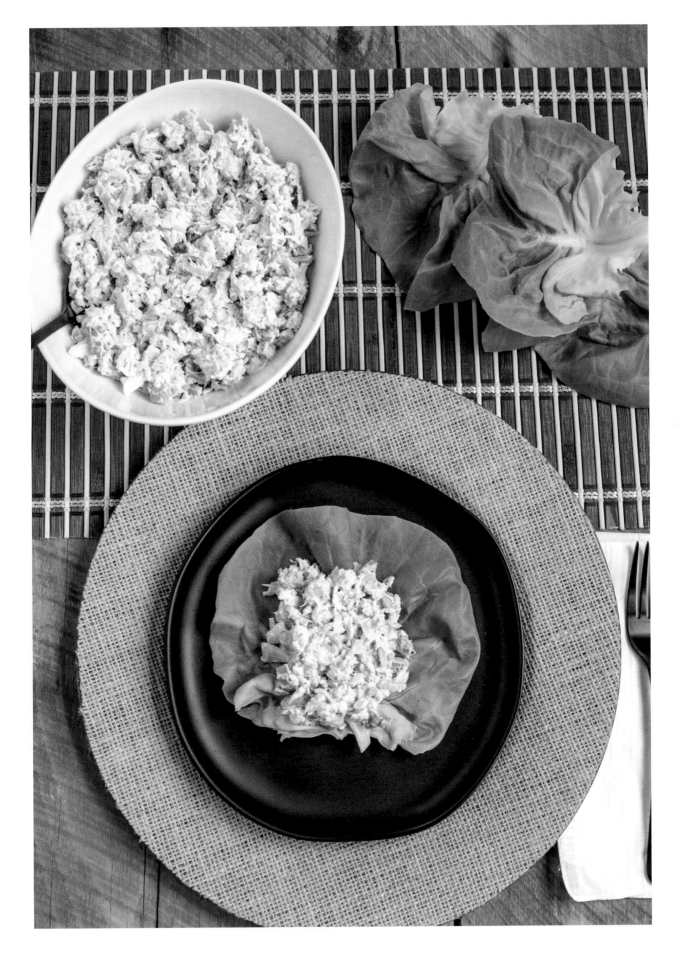

Cornbread Salad

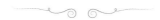

yield: 8 servings

prep time: 20 minutes (not including time to make cornbread), plus 2 hours to chill

1 recipe Skillet Cornbread (page 74), cooled

10 slices bacon, cooked and crumbled

2 medium tomatoes, seeded and diced

½ cup diced green bell peppers

1 green onion, sliced

1 cup mayonnaise

½ cup dill relish

½ cup dill pickle juice

⅛ teaspoon liquid stevia

Salt and ground black pepper

I just had to develop a cornbread salad for this book. You may not have heard of it before, but Grandma Ida Mae made it for every holiday and family gathering. We loved it! In my research, I found many different versions of cornbread salad. I kept mine as close to hers as I could.

1. Crumble the cornbread into bite-sized pieces and place in a large bowl. Put the bacon, tomatoes, green peppers, and green onion in the bowl with the cornbread and gently stir with a spoon.

2. In a small bowl, mix together the mayonnaise, relish, pickle juice, and stevia. Pour over the cornbread mixture and gently stir until well combined. Season to taste with salt and pepper.

3. Place the salad in the refrigerator to chill for at least 2 hours before serving. Leftovers can be stored in an airtight container in the refrigerator for up to 5 days.

NET CARBS 2.5g				
calories	fat	protein	carbs	fiber
424	34.4g	6.3g	4.7g	2.2g

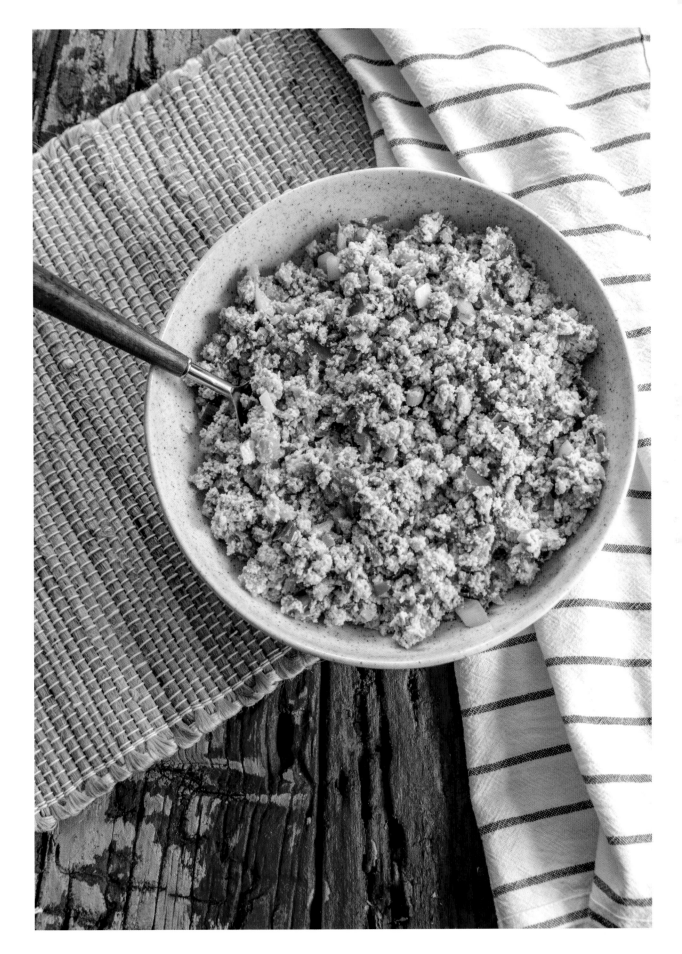

Spinach Salad with Hot Bacon Dressing

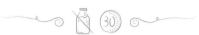

yield: 1 serving

prep time: 10 minutes

This is a great salad because it can easily be prepared for one person. And it's really pretty. You know looks matter to some people! The dressing is savory with a hint of sweetness.

1 loosely packed cup baby spinach leaves

1 hard-boiled egg, peeled and chopped

2 slices bacon, cooked and cut into small pieces

¼ cup raw pecan halves

6 fresh blackberries

DRESSING:

2 tablespoons hot bacon drippings

2 tablespoons white vinegar

1 tablespoon extra-virgin olive oil

1 tablespoon granular erythritol

1 teaspoon Dijon mustard

Salt and ground black pepper

1. Place the spinach leaves in a salad bowl. Top with the egg, bacon, pecans, and blackberries.

2. Prepare the dressing: In a small bowl, whisk together the bacon drippings, vinegar, olive oil, erythritol, and mustard. Season to taste with salt and pepper. Drizzle the dressing over the salad and serve immediately.

NET CARBS 1.7g				
calories	fat	protein	carbs	fiber
366	35.6g	8.5g	4.3g	2.6g

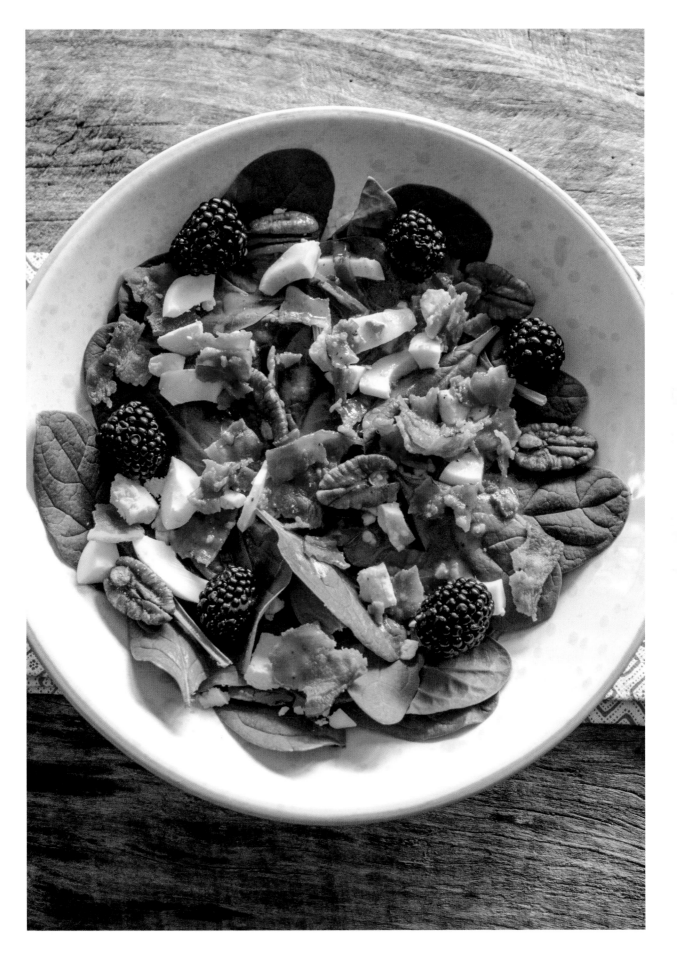

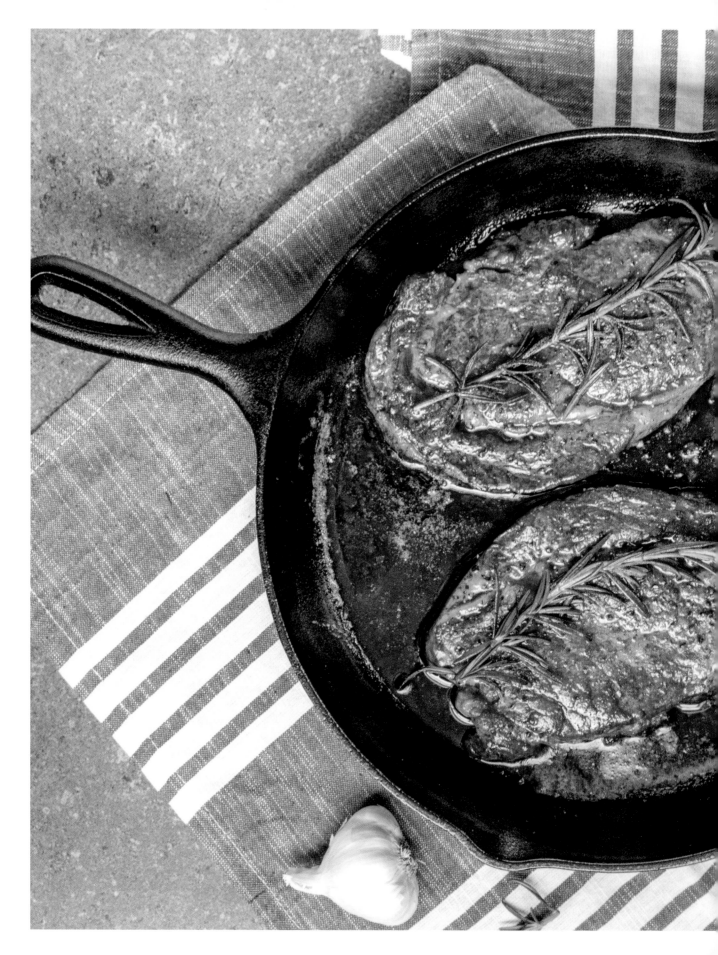

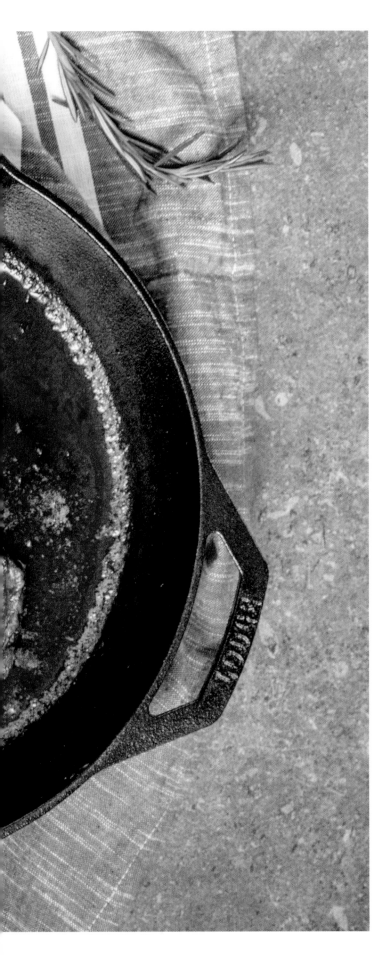

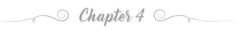
Chapter 4

Main Dishes

Open-Faced Sloppy Joes

yield: 6 servings
prep time: 10 minutes
cook time: 30 minutes

I grew up eating sloppy Joes on hamburger buns. For many years I used canned sloppy Joe sauce to make them. Homemade sloppy Joes are so much better! This is another one of those meals that makes great leftovers. The flavor develops and is even better the next day. I like to serve the meat over roasted spaghetti squash, but it's also great in a lettuce wrap.

2 pounds ground beef

1 clove garlic, minced

1 medium-sized green bell pepper, seeded and chopped

1 small onion, chopped

1 (8-ounce) can tomato paste

1 cup beef broth

2 tablespoons brown sugar substitute

2 tablespoons Worcestershire sauce

1 tablespoon prepared yellow mustard

Fresh flat-leaf parsley leaves, for garnish

1 recipe Roasted Spaghetti Squash (page 204), for serving (optional)

1. In a large skillet over medium heat, cook the ground beef with the garlic, green pepper, and onion, crumbling the meat with a large spoon as it cooks, until the meat is cooked through and no longer pink and the vegetables are tender, about 10 minutes. Drain the fat, if necessary.

2. Stir the tomato paste and broth into the ground beef mixture. When the paste is blended in, add the brown sugar substitute, Worcestershire sauce, and mustard and stir to combine. Simmer for 20 minutes to allow the flavors to meld.

3. Garnish with parsley leaves. If desired, serve over roasted spaghetti squash. Leftovers can be stored in an airtight container in the refrigerator for up to 5 days.

NET CARBS 3g				
calories	fat	protein	carbs	fiber
211	15.3g	14.1g	3.9g	0.9g

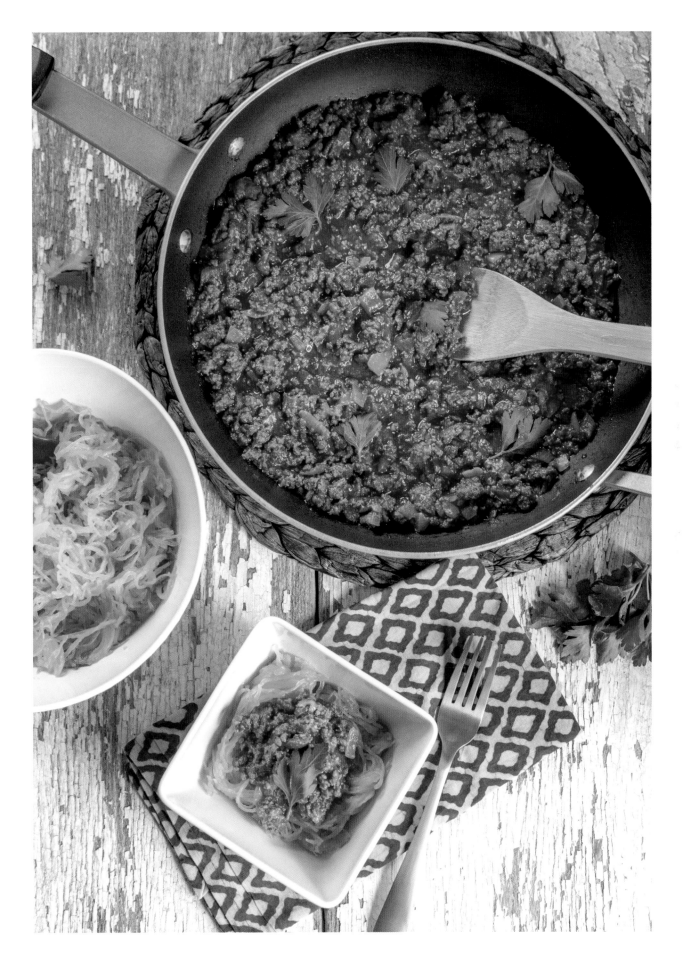

Memphis-Style Ribs

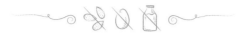

yield: 8 servings

prep time: 10 minutes (plus time to marinate, if desired)

cook time: 3 hours 30 minutes

2 full racks St. Louis-style spareribs (about 3 pounds each)

2 tablespoons avocado oil

1 recipe Tennessee Dry Rub (page 272)

You won't believe how easy it is to make fall-off-the-bone ribs at home! Don't let the cooking time deter you from making these ribs; they're worth it! My Tennessee Dry Rub gives them a smoky and slightly sweet flavor.

1. Preheat the oven to 275°F (unless you plan to marinate the ribs before baking them; see Step 4). Line a sheet pan with aluminum foil.

2. Pat the ribs dry. Use a knife to remove the thin membrane from the backside of the ribs. Don't skip this step; it is necessary to ensure that the ribs will be tender.

3. Brush the oil over both sides of the ribs. Sprinkle the dry rub evenly across both racks of ribs, then use your hands to rub it in on both sides. Place the ribs bone side down on the foil-lined pan.

4. If you have time, place the ribs in the refrigerator to marinate for at least 1 hour or up to 6 hours. If not, you can move on to the next step.

5. Bake the ribs for 3 hours 30 minutes, or until the meat is fall-off-the-bone tender. Leftovers can be stored in an airtight container in the refrigerator for up to 5 days.

NET CARBS 0.8g				
calories	fat	protein	carbs	fiber
371	31.9g	18.9g	1.6g	0.9g

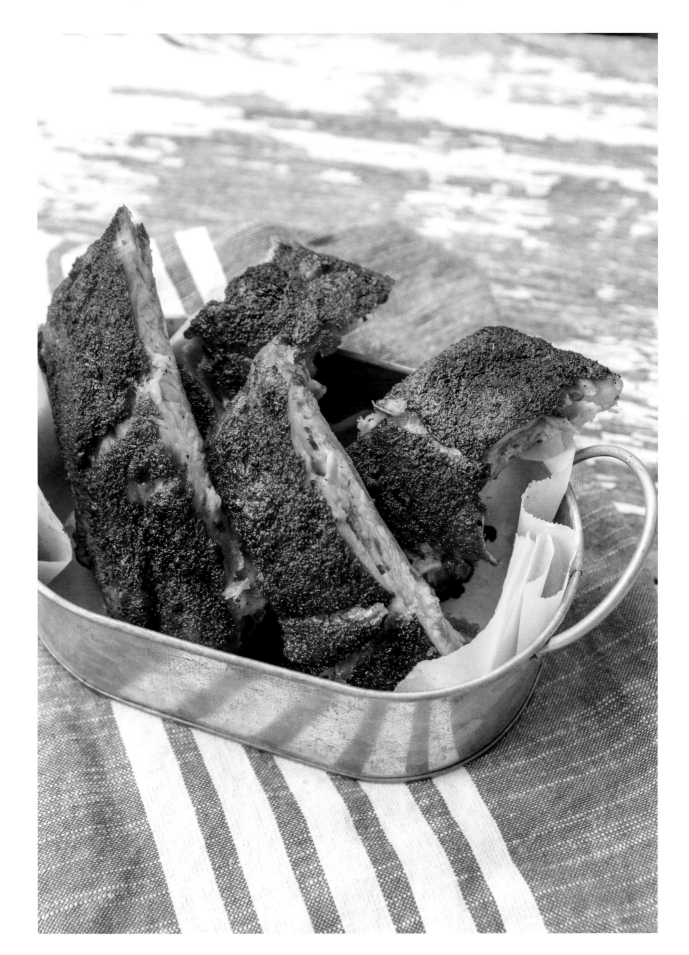

Shrimp Creole

yield: 6 servings

prep time: 10 minutes

cook time: 45 minutes

If you like spicy food, then you must try this recipe! My husband is a huge fan of Creole and Cajun cuisine. Whenever we visit a Gulf Coast town, he looks for dishes like this on the menu. Shrimp Creole is usually served over rice. Cauliflower rice is the perfect accompaniment to this keto version.

2 tablespoons salted butter

2 cloves garlic, minced

1 medium-sized green bell pepper, seeded and chopped

1 small white onion, chopped

1 rib celery, finely chopped

1 (28-ounce) can crushed tomatoes

1 cup vegetable broth

1 tablespoon Creole Seasoning (page 270)

1 tablespoon Worcestershire sauce

1 teaspoon hot sauce

1 bay leaf

1 teaspoon salt

½ teaspoon pepper

1 pound large shrimp, peeled and deveined

1½ recipes Basic Caulirice (page 202), for serving (optional)

Fresh flat-leaf parsley leaves, for garnish (optional)

Sliced green onions, for garnish (optional)

1. Melt the butter in a stockpot over medium heat. Add the garlic, green pepper, onion, and celery and cook, stirring occasionally, until the vegetables are tender and the onion is translucent.

2. Stir in the tomatoes, broth, Creole seasoning, Worcestershire sauce, hot sauce, and bay leaf. Season with the salt and pepper. Bring the mixture to a boil, then reduce the heat and simmer for 30 minutes.

3. Add the shrimp to the pot and continue cooking until the shrimp is just cooked and has turned pink, 4 to 5 minutes.

4. Remove the bay leaf. If desired, serve over caulirice and garnish with parsley and sliced green onions. Leftovers can be stored in an airtight container in the refrigerator for up to 5 days.

Note:

I purchased peeled and deveined shrimp to make this dish. If you're using shrimp with the peels on, allow for more prep time.

NET CARBS 9g				
calories	fat	protein	carbs	fiber
141	4.5g	13.7g	11.9g	3g

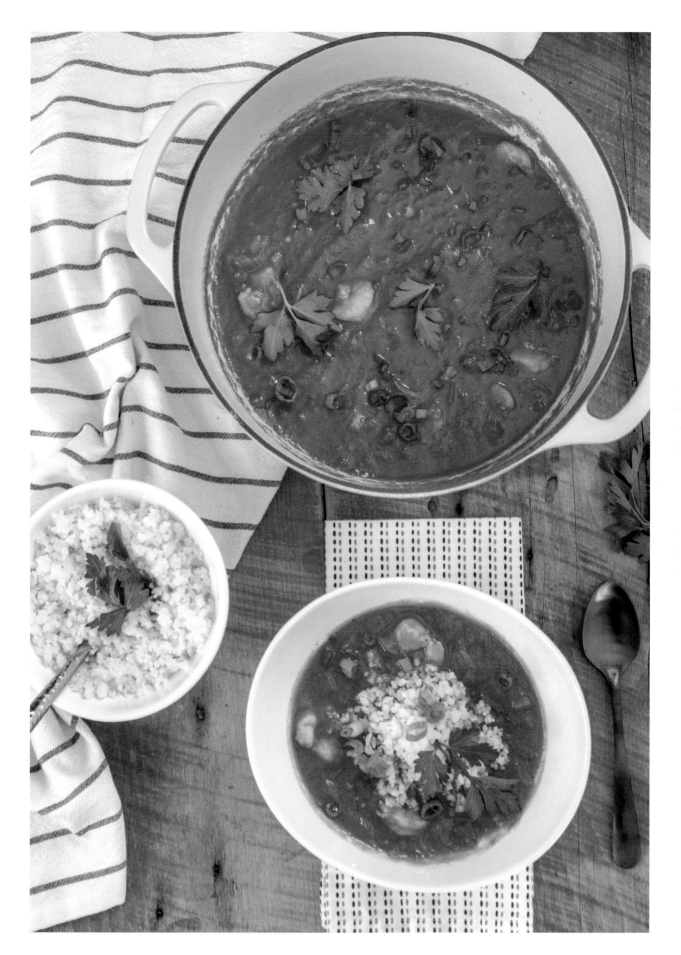

Chili Cheese Pot Pie

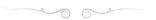

yield: 6 servings

prep time: 15 minutes

cook time: 45 minutes

This is comfort food at its best! I'm biased toward recipes that are topped with some sort of biscuit. Two things my family loves are chili and biscuits. With my cheesy low-carb biscuits, this pot pie is a match made in heaven!

FILLING:

2 pounds ground beef

½ cup diced onions, or 2 tablespoons dried minced onions

2 cloves garlic, minced

1 (14½-ounce) can petite diced tomatoes

1½ tablespoons chili powder

2 teaspoons ground cumin

1 teaspoon smoked paprika

BISCUIT TOPPING:

1½ cups finely ground blanched almond flour

2 teaspoons baking powder

½ teaspoon garlic powder

¼ teaspoon salt

½ cup shredded cheddar cheese

¼ cup sour cream

2 large eggs

2 tablespoons salted butter, melted but not hot

1. Make the filling: In a 12-inch cast-iron skillet or other ovenproof skillet, cook the ground beef with the onions and garlic over medium heat, crumbling the meat with a large spoon as it cooks, until the meat is browned and the onions and garlic are translucent, about 10 minutes. Drain the fat, if necessary.

2. Stir in the tomatoes and seasonings. Simmer over low heat for 15 minutes, then remove from the heat.

3. Preheat the oven to 375°F.

4. Make the biscuit topping: In a bowl, whisk together the almond flour, baking powder, garlic powder, and salt until well combined. In a separate bowl, stir together the cheese, sour cream, eggs, and melted butter. Add the wet ingredients to the dry ingredients and gently stir until well combined.

5. Drop the biscuit topping mixture by the large spoonful onto the chili beef mixture in the skillet.

6. Bake for 20 minutes or until the biscuits are cooked through and browned on top. Leftovers can be stored in an airtight container in the refrigerator for up to 5 days.

NET CARBS 6.7g				
calories	fat	protein	carbs	fiber
477	37.3g	23.6g	10.3g	4.3g

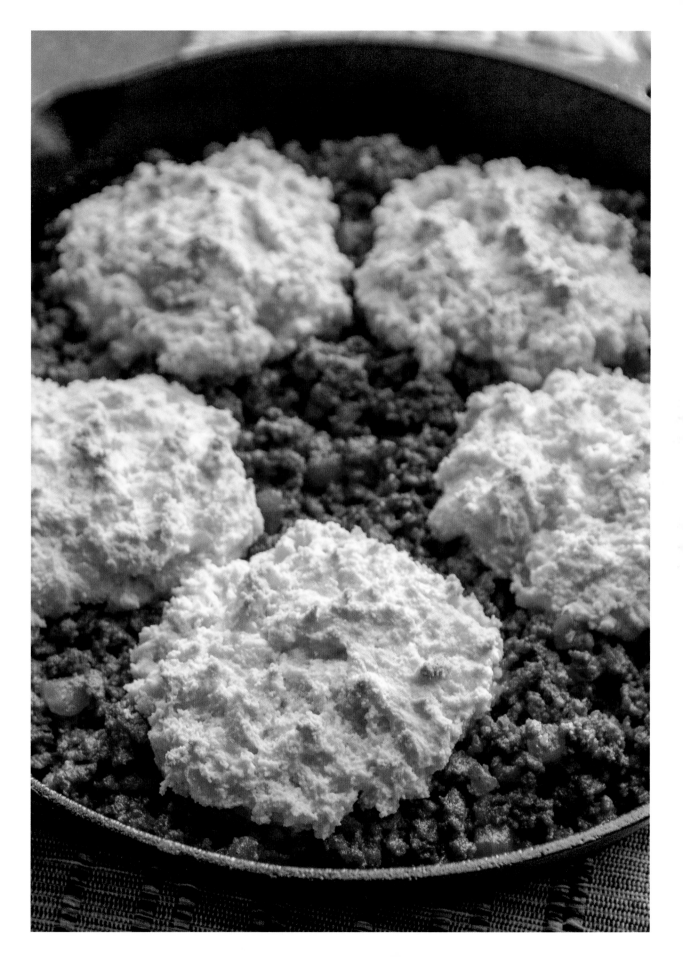

Slow Cooker Pulled Pork

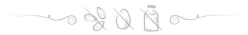

yield: 10 servings

prep time: 10 minutes

cook time: 3 to 4 hours

1 (5-pound) bone-in pork butt or shoulder roast

¼ cup Tennessee Dry Rub (page 272)

1 medium onion, thinly sliced

4 cloves garlic, peeled

1 cup apple cider vinegar

¼ cup water

Who doesn't love a good slow cooker meal? What I like about pulled pork is all the different ways you can use it: in lettuce wraps, on salads, and even on Barbecue Pulled Pork Pizza (page 184). The possibilities are endless!

1. Trim the excess fat from the pork roast. Pat the meat dry and season on all sides with the dry rub, massaging the seasoning into the meat.

2. Lay the onion slices and garlic cloves evenly in a large slow cooker. Pour in the vinegar and water. Gently place the pork in the slow cooker.

3. Cover and cook on high for 3 to 4 hours or on low for 6 to 8 hours, until the meat is cooked through and easily falls apart when pierced with a fork.

4. Use two forks to shred the pork before serving. Leftovers can be stored in an airtight container in the refrigerator for up to 5 days.

Note:

You can drizzle some of the leftover drippings over the shredded pork to add more flavor and keep it moist.

NET CARBS 0.5g				
calories	fat	protein	carbs	fiber
530	30g	60.4g	0.3g	0.2g

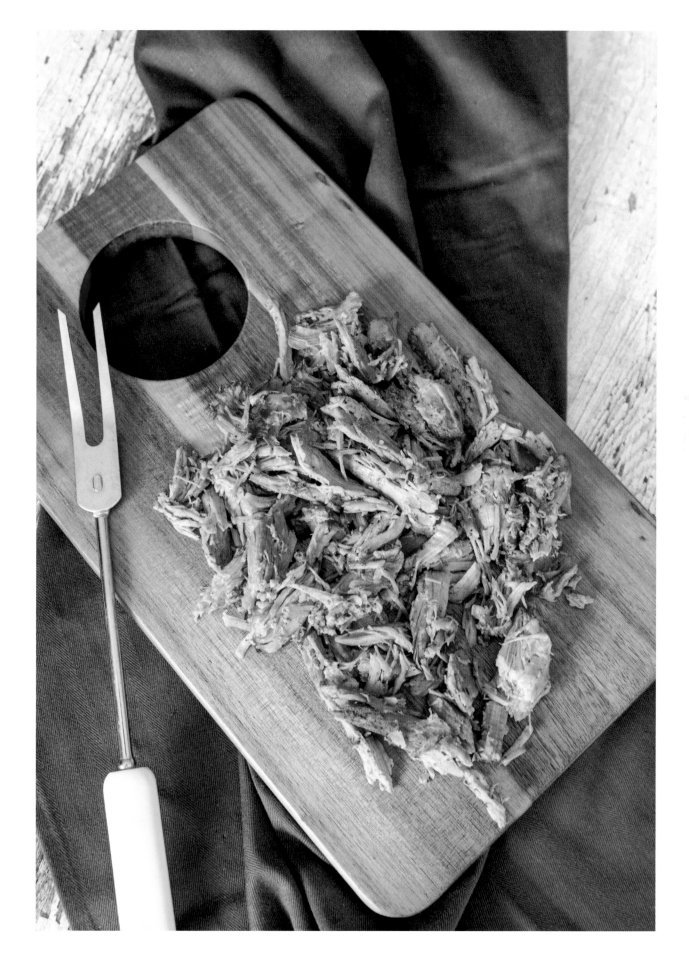

Crispy Chicken Wings

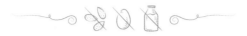

yield: 4 servings

prep time: 10 minutes

cook time: 1 hour 15 minutes

If I had to choose one food that my family consistently orders out but also loves to eat at home, it would be chicken wings. We always order them naked and eat them with ranch dressing. But at home, where I know exactly what's going into my food, I lightly season them, as in this recipe. This low and slow baking method, with a bit of baking powder thrown into the seasoning mix, might be a little different from how you normally make wings, but I encourage you to try it. It gives the wings extra-crispy skin! These wings are great served with my homemade Ranch Dressing (page 274) and/or Buffalo Sauce (page 275).

1 pound chicken wings

1 tablespoon baking powder

1 teaspoon salt

½ teaspoon paprika

¼ teaspoon cayenne pepper (optional)

¼ teaspoon ground black pepper

1. Place an oven rack in the lowest position and another rack in the highest position. Preheat the oven to 250°F. Line a sheet pan with parchment paper.

2. Pat the chicken wings dry. Put the rest of the ingredients in a gallon-sized resealable plastic bag. Place the wings in the bag, seal the top, and shake until the wings are lightly coated all over. Spread the wings evenly on the lined pan.

3. Put the wings on the lower rack of the oven and bake for 30 minutes. Increase the oven temperature to 425°F, move the wings to the upper rack, and bake for 45 more minutes or until golden brown. Serve immediately.

NET CARBS 0.9g				
calories	fat	protein	carbs	fiber
222	14.6g	19.9g	1.1g	0.2g

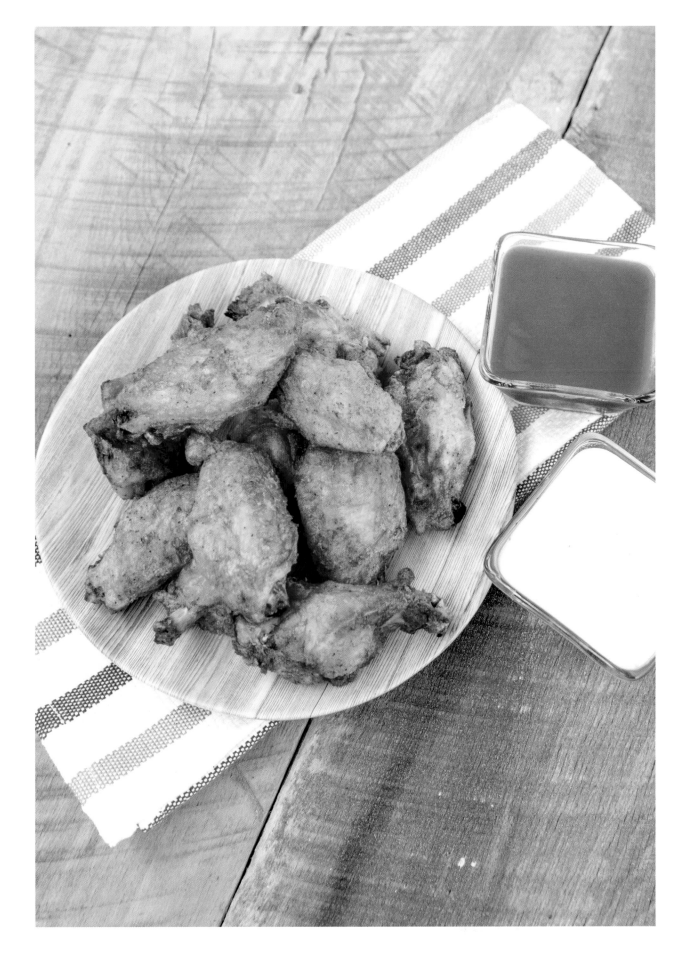

Cheeseburger "Mac" Helper

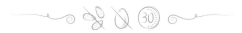

yield: 4 servings

prep time: 5 minutes

cook time: 20 or 40 minutes

This dish isn't fancy, but it sure is flavorful and quick to prepare on a busy weeknight! Growing up, I ate a lot of Hamburger Helper meals. When I first got married, I gravitated to those easy prepackaged solutions. I'm glad I now know that it's just as easy to prepare your own—and much healthier!

1 pound ground beef

½ cup chopped onions, or 2 tablespoons dried minced onions

2 teaspoons paprika

1 teaspoon chili powder

1 teaspoon garlic powder

1 teaspoon dried parsley

½ teaspoon salt

½ teaspoon ground black pepper

1 (8-ounce) can tomato sauce

1 (12-ounce) bag frozen cauliflower florets

2 cups shredded cheddar cheese

Fresh flat-leaf parsley, for garnish (optional)

1. In a large skillet over medium heat, cook the ground beef with the onions, crumbling the meat with a large spoon as it cooks, until the meat is browned and the onions are translucent, about 10 minutes. Drain the fat, if necessary.

2. Stir in the paprika, chili powder, garlic powder, parsley, salt, pepper, and tomato sauce and simmer for 5 minutes.

3. Stir in the cauliflower, cover, and continue cooking, stirring occasionally, until the cauliflower is tender.

4. Stir in the cheese and serve immediately, or reduce the heat to low and simmer for an additional 20 minutes for more depth of flavor, then stir in the cheese. Garnish with parsley, if desired. Leftovers can be stored in an airtight container in the refrigerator for up to 5 days.

NET CARBS 5.8g				
calories	fat	protein	carbs	fiber
381	28g	23.5g	8.5g	2.7g

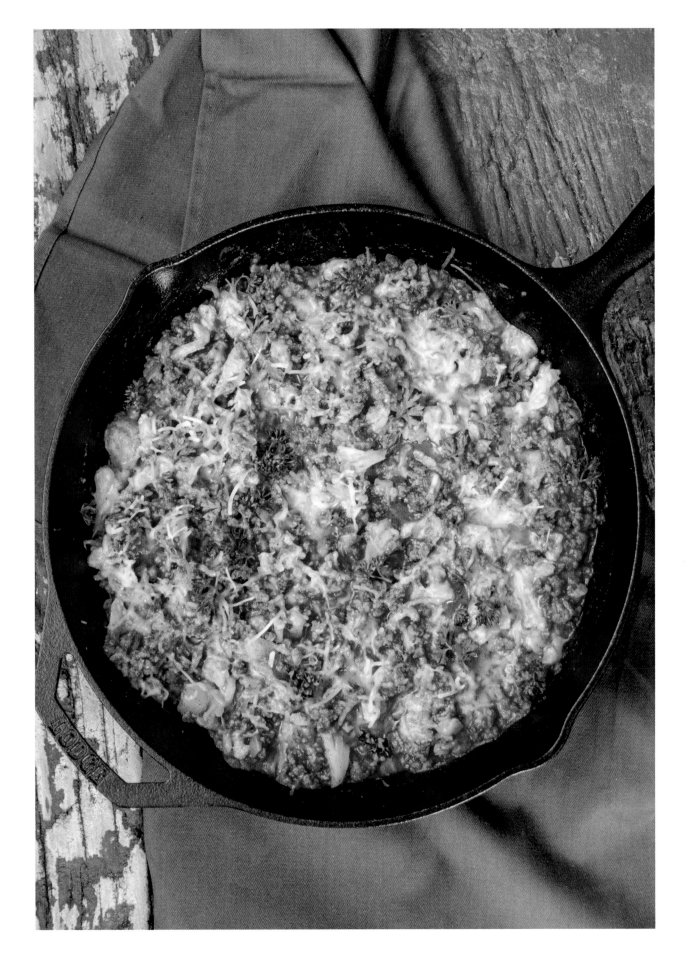

Creamy Broccoli and Ground Beef Casserole

yield: 6 servings
prep time: 10 minutes
cook time: 30 minutes

This Southern girl loves casseroles! This dish is a favorite around here for sure. How can you go wrong with a casserole that has a creamy cheese-laden white sauce in it?

1½ pounds ground beef

½ cup chopped onions

1 clove garlic, minced

1 (16-ounce) bag frozen broccoli

1 (8-ounce) package cream cheese

½ cup heavy whipping cream

½ cup grated Parmesan cheese

Salt and ground black pepper

1 cup shredded mozzarella cheese

½ teaspoon red pepper flakes (optional)

1. Preheat the oven to 375°F and grease a 9 by 13-inch baking dish.

2. In a medium-sized skillet over medium heat, cook the ground beef with the onions and garlic, crumbling the meat with a large spoon as it cooks, until the meat is browned and the onions are translucent, about 10 minutes. Drain the fat, if necessary. Set aside.

3. Cook the broccoli according to the package directions, then drain well.

4. Meanwhile, make the sauce: Place the cream cheese, heavy cream, and Parmesan cheese in a small saucepan over low heat and stir continuously until melted and blended. Season to taste with salt and pepper.

5. In a large bowl, gently stir together the beef mixture, broccoli, and sauce. Spread this mixture in the greased baking dish and top evenly with the mozzarella cheese and red pepper flakes, if using.

6. Bake for 15 to 20 minutes, until the cheese is melted and the top is lightly browned. Leftovers can be stored in an airtight container in the refrigerator for up to 5 days.

NET CARBS 4.5g				
calories	fat	protein	carbs	fiber
605	47.3g	37g	7g	2.5g

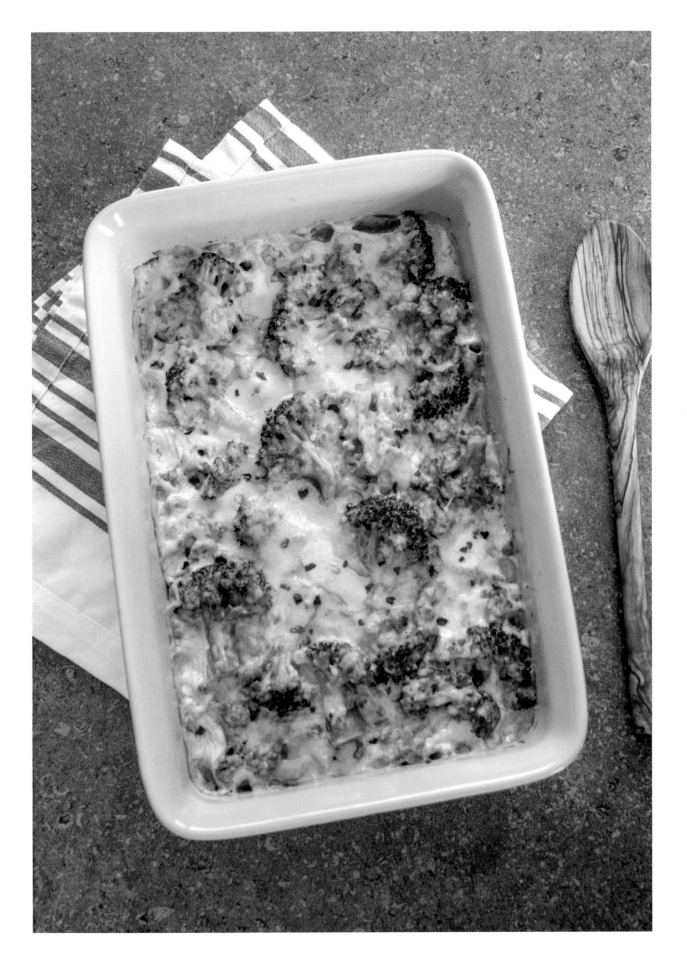

Bacon Cheeseburger Mini Meatloaves

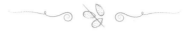

yield: 8 mini meatloaves
(2 per serving)

prep time: 15 minutes

cook time: 30 minutes

Meatloaf wasn't my favorite growing up, but it grew on me as I got older. Now I love it! Most people who eat low-carb stay away from meatloaf because it usually contains breadcrumbs. These little breadcrumb-free meatloaves are so yummy, and they're wrapped in bacon, too, so there!

8 slices bacon, partially cooked (see Notes)

1 pound ground beef

1 cup shredded cheddar cheese

1 large egg

½ cup sugar-free ketchup, plus extra for the tops

¼ cup chopped dill pickles

2 tablespoons dried minced onions

1 tablespoon Worcestershire sauce

¼ teaspoon salt

½ teaspoon ground black pepper

1. Preheat the oven to 375°F. Grease 8 wells of a standard-size 12-well muffin pan or line with parchment paper.

2. Wrap a slice of partially cooked bacon around the side of each prepared muffin well.

3. Place the rest of the ingredients in a large bowl. Use your hands to combine the ingredients until just blended, being careful not to overmix.

4. Divide the meat mixture evenly among the bacon-lined wells of the muffin pan, filling each well to the top of the bacon. Brush the tops of the meatloaves with ketchup.

5. Bake for 30 minutes or until a meat thermometer registers 160°F when inserted in the middle of a meatloaf. Leftovers can be stored in an airtight container in the refrigerator for up to 5 days.

Notes:

The bacon should be cooked just long enough that it releases some of its fat (so that you don't end up with meatloaves sitting in pools of bacon drippings) but remains bendy; do not cook the bacon until it's crispy.

You can use a stand mixer fitted with a dough hook on low speed to make mixing easier.

NET CARBS 4.8g				
calories	fat	protein	carbs	fiber
548	42.3g	34.8g	5.2g	0.4g

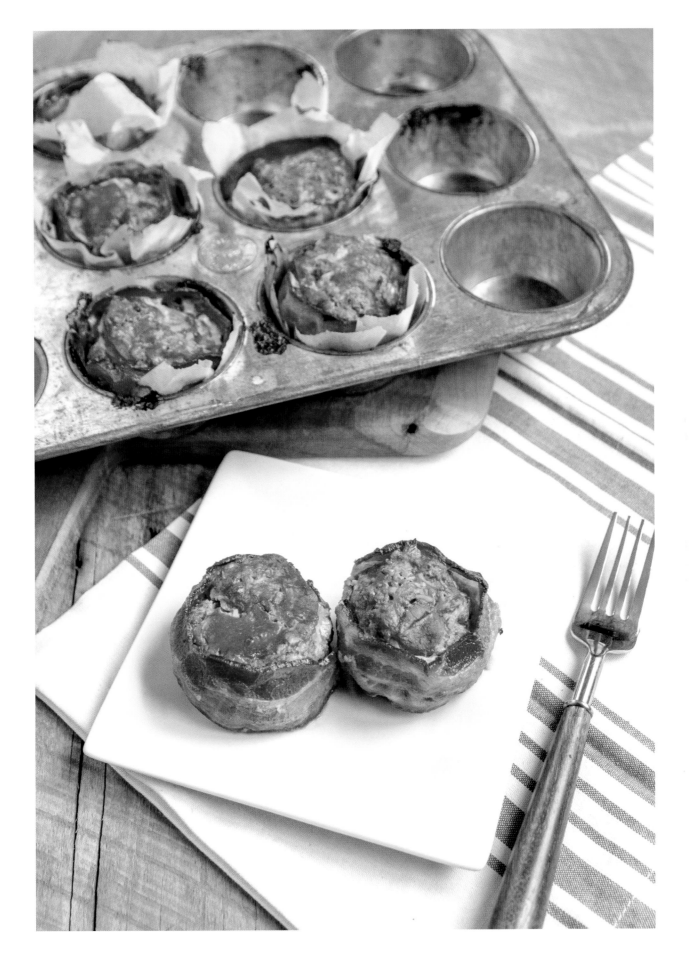

Sheet Pan Garlic Butter Shrimp

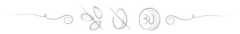

yield: 4 servings

prep time: 10 minutes

cook time: 10 minutes

1½ pounds medium shrimp, peeled and deveined

½ cup (1 stick) salted butter, melted

¼ cup chopped fresh flat-leaf parsley

2 cloves garlic, minced

Pinch of salt

Pinch of ground black pepper

1 lemon, sliced

Sometimes you need a fast meal, but you still want it to taste great, right? It doesn't get any easier than this garlic butter shrimp. It's great served with a salad or on top of my Easy Caulimash (page 210) or Basic Caulirice (page 202).

1. Preheat the oven to 400°F. Line a sheet pan with parchment paper.

2. Pat the shrimp dry. Arrange the shrimp in a single layer on the lined pan.

3. In a small bowl, stir together the melted butter, parsley, garlic, salt, and pepper. Pour the butter mixture evenly over the shrimp. Place the lemon slices on top of the shrimp. Bake for 8 to 10 minutes, until the shrimp is pink and opaque. Serve immediately.

Note:

I purchased peeled and deveined shrimp to make this dish. If you're using shrimp with the peels on, allow for more prep time.

NET CARBS 1.4g				
calories	fat	protein	carbs	fiber
320	24.4g	25g	1.7g	0.3g

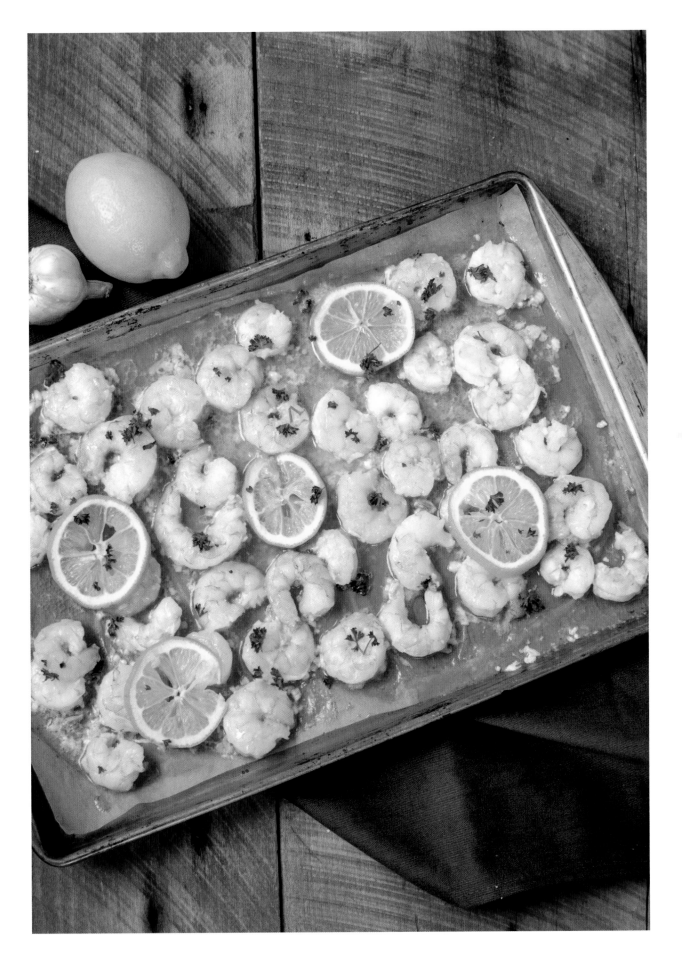

Ground Beef Stroganoff

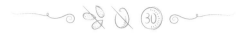

yield: 6 servings

prep time: 10 minutes

cook time: 20 minutes

Beef Stroganoff is comfort food to me because I grew up eating it. But it's another one of those meals that I used to make from a box. (You must be thinking, how did she ever learn to cook?!) That boxed stuff doesn't even compare with this rich and creamy Stroganoff. It's so good served on top of my Easy Caulimash (page 210), as pictured.

1½ pounds ground beef

½ cup finely chopped onions

2 cloves garlic, minced

4 ounces white mushrooms, sliced

4 ounces cream cheese (½ cup), softened

1 cup beef broth

¼ cup heavy whipping cream

¼ cup water

1 tablespoon Worcestershire sauce

Salt and ground black pepper

½ cup sour cream

1. In a large skillet over medium heat, cook the ground beef with the onions, garlic, and mushrooms, crumbling the meat with a large spoon it as cooks, until the meat is browned and the onions are softened and translucent, about 10 minutes. Drain the fat, if necessary.

2. Stir in the cream cheese and cook until melted. Add the broth, cream, water, and Worcestershire sauce and stir to combine. Continue to simmer for 5 minutes.

3. Season to taste with salt and pepper. Stir in the sour cream and serve. Leftovers can be stored in an airtight container in the refrigerator for up to 5 days.

NET CARBS 2.4g				
calories	fat	protein	carbs	fiber
396	31.6g	22.4g	2.8g	0.4g

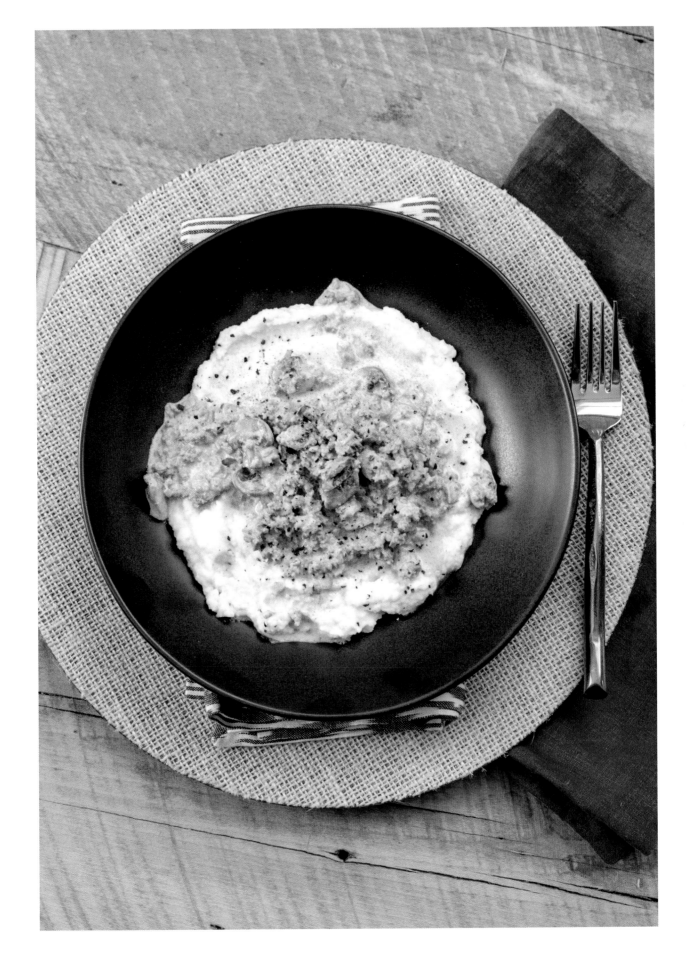

Southern Fish Fry

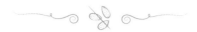

yield: 4 servings
prep time: 20 minutes
cook time: 20 minutes

You need something to go with those Hushpuppies (page 98), right? Fried fish and hushpuppies were made for one another. I think it's time for a fish fry! You can find my sample menu on page 47.

High-quality oil, for frying

1 pound white fish fillets

½ cup finely crushed pork rinds

½ cup grated Parmesan cheese

1 large egg

2 tablespoons heavy whipping cream

FOR SERVING:

Lemon wedges

½ cup Tartar Sauce (page 276)

SPECIAL EQUIPMENT:
Candy thermometer

1. Attach a candy thermometer to a Dutch oven or other large heavy pot, then pour in 3 inches of oil and set the pot over medium-high heat. Heat the oil to 350°F.

2. While the oil is heating, pat the fish dry and set aside. In a shallow dish, combine the pork rinds and Parmesan cheese. In another shallow dish, whisk together the egg and cream.

3. Dip a fish fillet into the egg mixture and coat both sides, allowing the excess to drip back into the bowl. Gently press the pork rind mixture onto both sides of the fish. Repeat with the remaining fillets. Refrigerate the breaded fish for 10 minutes.

4. Working in small batches, fry the fish for about 2 minutes per side, until the outside is golden brown and the inside is opaque and flaky. Serve immediately with lemon wedges and tartar sauce.

NET CARBS 0.6g				
calories	fat	protein	carbs	fiber
213	8.4g	30g	0.6g	0g

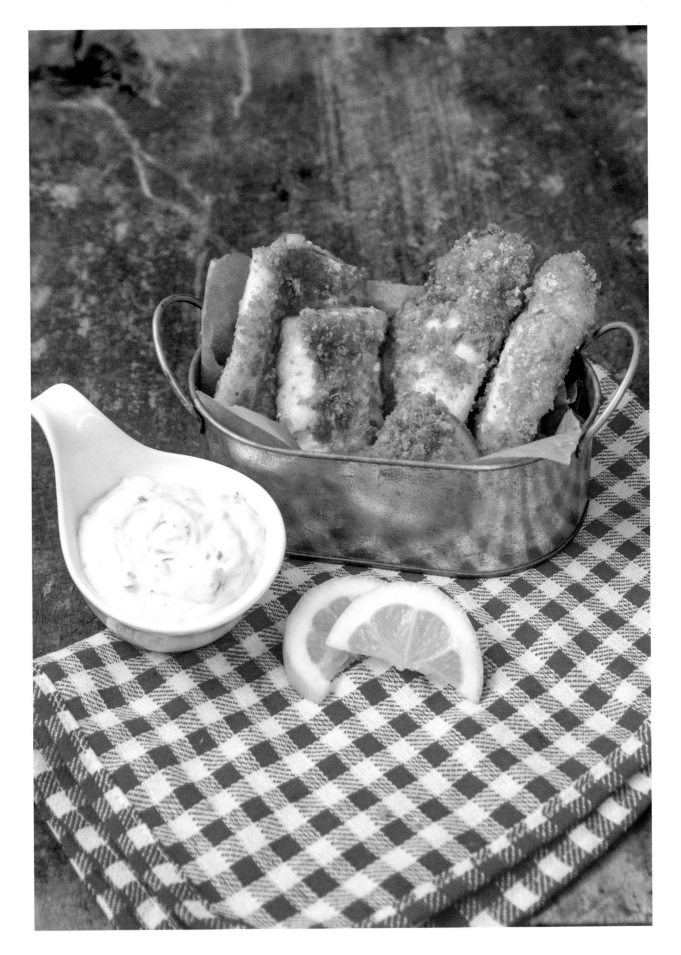

Barbecue Chicken Drumsticks

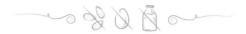

yield: 4 servings

prep time: 5 minutes

cook time: 1 hour

10 to 12 large chicken drumsticks (about 1 pound)

Salt

1 cup Easy BBQ Sauce (page 277), divided

My family thinks these drumsticks are finger-licking good! You can use store-bought sugar-free barbecue sauce, but they're really yummy when made with my homemade barbecue sauce.

1. Preheat the oven to 400°F. Line a sheet pan with parchment paper.

2. Place the drumsticks in a single layer on the lined sheet pan. Lightly sprinkle both sides of the chicken with salt, then brush both sides with ½ cup of the BBQ sauce.

3. Bake for 30 minutes, then remove from the oven, turn the chicken over, and brush the chicken with the remaining ½ cup of BBQ sauce. Return to the oven and bake for 30 more minutes or until cooked through. To determine doneness, pierce the meat to the bone; if the juices run clear, it's done.

4. For crispier skin, turn the oven to broil and broil the chicken for 1 to 2 minutes, watching carefully so that it doesn't burn. Serve immediately. Leftovers can be stored in an airtight container in the refrigerator for up to 5 days.

NET CARBS 0.5g				
calories	fat	protein	carbs	fiber
186	10.4g	20.7g	0.8g	0g

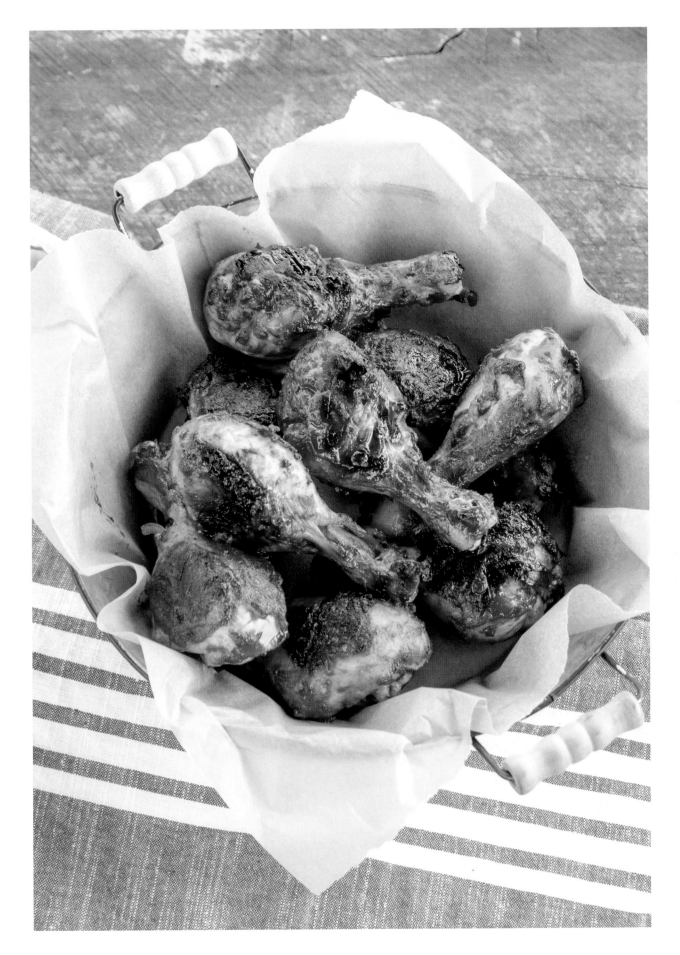

Reverse Sear Garlic Rosemary Rib-Eye Steaks

yield: 2 servings

prep time: 5 minutes, plus 30 minutes for the steaks to come to room temperature and 15 minutes to rest

cook time: 27 minutes

We are blessed to have an abundance of grass-fed beef that is raised locally by friends of ours. This preparation method has you slow-cook the steaks in the oven before finishing them off with a hot sear. Reverse searing creates wonderfully juicy medium-rare meat, and it's my family's favorite way to eat steak. The extra time it takes to cook steaks this way is worth it. The herbed browned butter spooned over the top makes this dish extra decadent.

2 (6-ounce) bone-in rib-eye steaks (1½ inches thick)

Salt and ground black pepper

2 tablespoons salted butter

2 fresh rosemary sprigs

2 cloves garlic, minced

1. Take the steaks out of the refrigerator. Generously salt and pepper both sides of the steaks. Allow to sit at room temperature for 30 minutes.

2. Preheat the oven to 275°F. Line a sheet pan with foil and place a wire cooling rack on top.

3. Place the steaks on the rack on top of the foil-lined pan. Bake for 25 minutes or until the internal temperature of the meat reaches 125°F. Remove from the oven and let rest for 15 minutes.

4. Preheat a cast-iron skillet over medium-high heat. Put the butter in the hot pan; it will melt quickly. Place the steaks in the skillet and hard sear the first side for 1 minute (see Note), then flip the steaks. Add the rosemary and garlic to the pan and swirl it around. Hard sear the steaks for 1 more minute, tilting the pan to spoon the melted butter and herbs over them. Serve immediately.

Note:

A hard sear involves cooking meat at a high temperature to form a crust while cooking the inside as little as possible. Use a cast-iron skillet for best results.

NET CARBS 1.9g				
calories	fat	protein	carbs	fiber
559	46g	32.8g	3.9g	2.1g

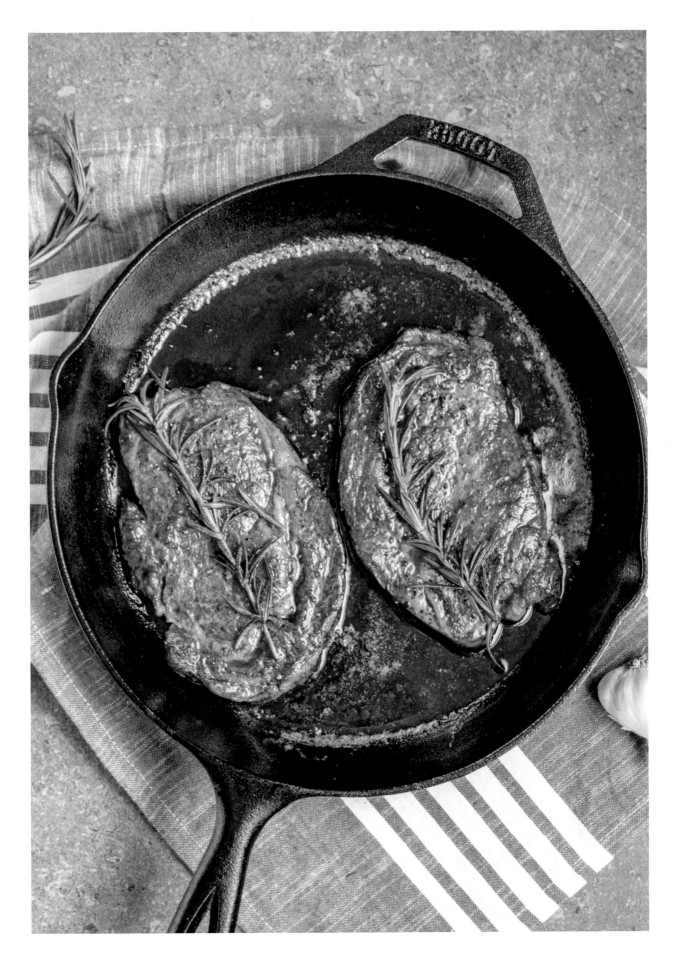

Cajun Sausage and Rice

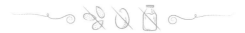

yield: 4 servings

prep time: 10 minutes

cook time: 25 minutes

If you enjoy spicy food, then this dish is for you! It's one of my husband's favorites. So easy to prepare, it makes a great weeknight meal.

2 tablespoons avocado oil

14 ounces fully cooked andouille sausage, sliced

½ cup diced onions

½ cup diced green bell peppers

1 rib celery, diced

1 (12-ounce) bag frozen riced cauliflower

1 cup vegetable broth

1 teaspoon Creole Seasoning (page 270)

1 bay leaf

1. Heat the oil in a large, deep skillet over medium heat. Brown the sausage for 2 to 3 minutes. Add the onions, green peppers, and celery to the skillet and cook until the vegetables are tender and the onions are translucent.

2. Add the cauliflower, broth, Creole seasoning, and bay leaf to the skillet. Continue cooking, stirring occasionally, until the cauliflower is tender.

3. Reduce the heat to low and simmer for 10 more minutes, until the mixture is slightly thickened. Remove the bay leaf before serving.

NET CARBS 4g				
calories	fat	protein	carbs	fiber
308	25g	16.5g	6.8g	2.8g

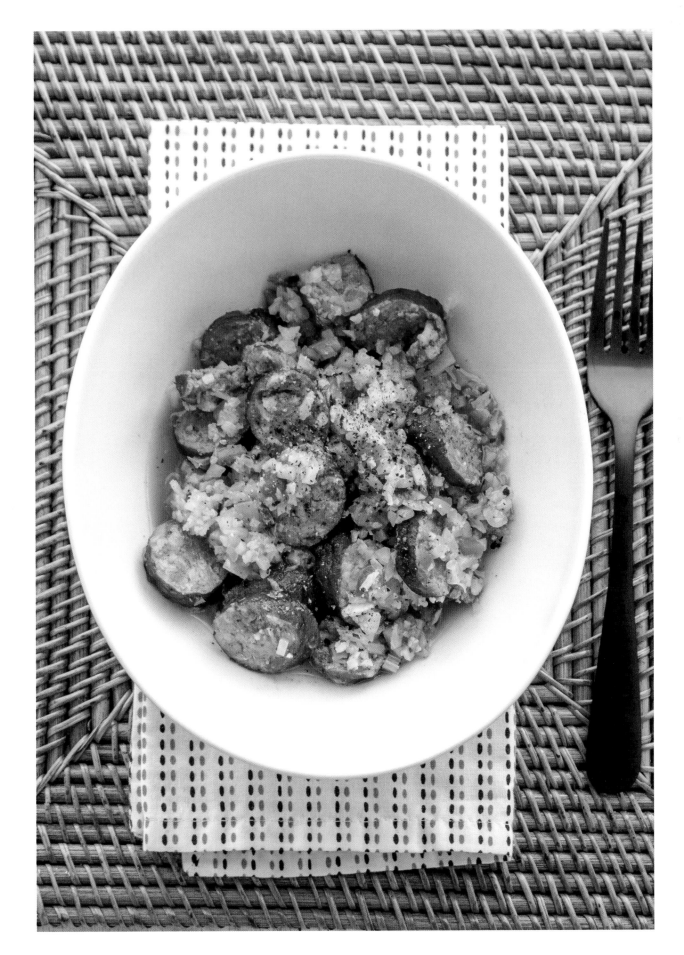

Slow Cooker Bourbon Chicken

yield: 4 servings

prep time: 10 minutes

cook time: 2 to 3 hours

1 pound chicken tenderloins

2 cloves garlic, minced

¼ cup gluten-free soy sauce

¼ cup bourbon

¼ cup sugar-free ketchup

¼ cup brown sugar substitute

1 tablespoon apple cider vinegar

1 teaspoon ginger powder

½ teaspoon xanthan gum (see Note)

1 recipe Basic Caulirice (page 202), for serving (optional)

Sliced green onions, for garnish (optional)

Bring a taste of the South to your table with this spirited chicken dish. It's sweet and savory, and the best part is how easy it is to make!

1. Grease the inside of a slow cooker with oil. Place the chicken in the slow cooker.

2. In a small bowl, combine the garlic, soy sauce, bourbon, ketchup, brown sugar substitute, vinegar, and ginger powder. Stir to blend well. Pour the mixture evenly over the chicken.

3. Place the lid on the slow cooker and cook on low for 2 to 3 hours, until the chicken is no longer pink in the center. Remove the chicken from the slow cooker and shred with two forks.

4. If using the xanthan gum, stir it into the juices in the slow cooker. Turn the slow cooker up to high for 5 minutes and stir frequently until the sauce has thickened.

5. Return the chicken to the slow cooker and stir to coat the meat in the sauce. Serve over caulirice and garnish with sliced green onions, if desired.

Note:

If you don't have xanthan gum on hand, you can leave it out. It won't affect the flavor of the dish; it just acts as a thickener for the juices.

NET CARBS 2.5g				
calories	fat	protein	carbs	fiber
144	0g	24.3g	3g	0.5g

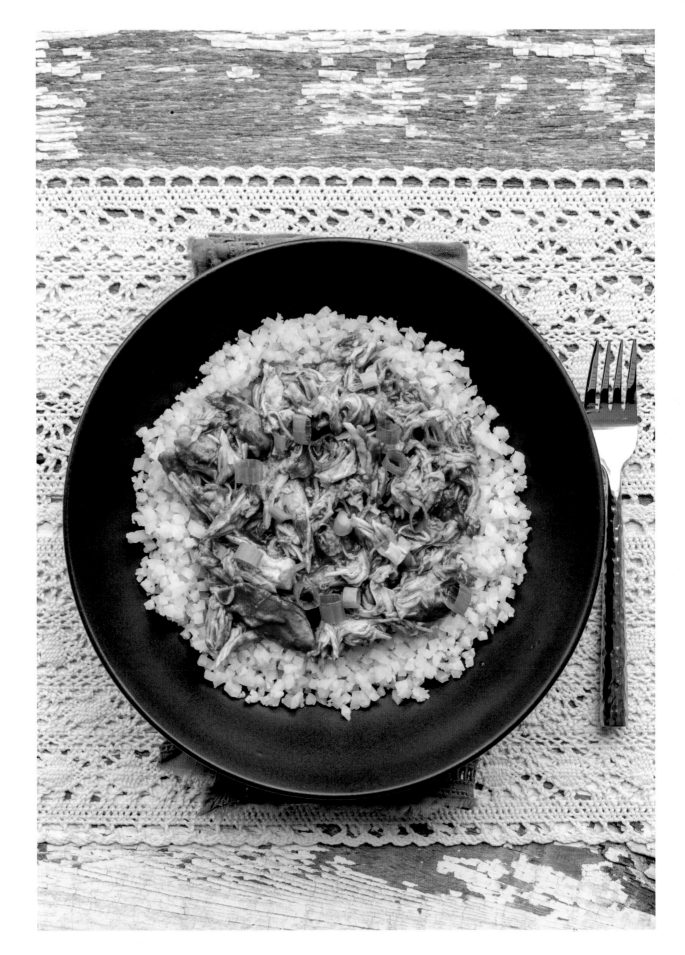

Fried Chicken

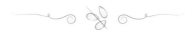

yield: 4 servings

prep time: 15 minutes

cook time: 35 minutes

Is there anything more Southern than fried chicken? I grew up in Kentucky, and that's where the world-famous fried chicken restaurant chain originated. (A little reminder: KFC stands for Kentucky Fried Chicken.) The truth is, however, that most Southerners I know prefer fried chicken from a regional chain called Lee's Famous Recipe; it is fried chicken from Lee's, not KFC, that shows up at potlucks and impromptu family gatherings. All my family members love my low-carb recipe, by the way, including my very picky son. You might have thought that you couldn't have fried chicken on keto, but this recipe will change your mind!

High-quality oil, for frying

2 large eggs

¼ cup heavy whipping cream

¼ cup water

1 cup whey protein powder (unflavored and unsweetened)

1 tablespoon paprika

1 teaspoon ground black pepper

1 teaspoon garlic powder

1 teaspoon onion powder

1 teaspoon salt

4 bone-in, skin-on chicken breast halves or thighs, or 8 drumsticks (1¾ to 2¾ pounds)

SPECIAL EQUIPMENT:

Candy thermometer

1. Attach a candy thermometer to a Dutch oven or other large heavy pot, then pour in 3 inches of oil and set the pot over medium-high heat. Heat the oil to 350°F.

2. While the oil is heating, beat the eggs, cream, and water together in a shallow dish.

3. Put the whey powder, spices, and salt in a gallon-sized resealable plastic bag. Seal and gently shake.

4. Dip both sides of a chicken piece in the egg mixture, allowing the excess to drip back into the bowl, then place the chicken in the bag with the spice mixture. Repeat with one or two more pieces of chicken, depending on the size of the pieces. Seal the bag and gently shake to coat the chicken. Repeat until all the chicken pieces are coated.

5. Working in small batches, fry the chicken, turning with tongs every 1 to 2 minutes, until the skin is deep golden brown and a meat thermometer inserted into the thickest part of the chicken registers 165°F, 10 to 12 minutes. Use the tongs to remove the chicken from the pot and transfer it to a wire rack. Repeat with the remaining chicken. Allow the fried chicken to rest for 10 minutes before serving.

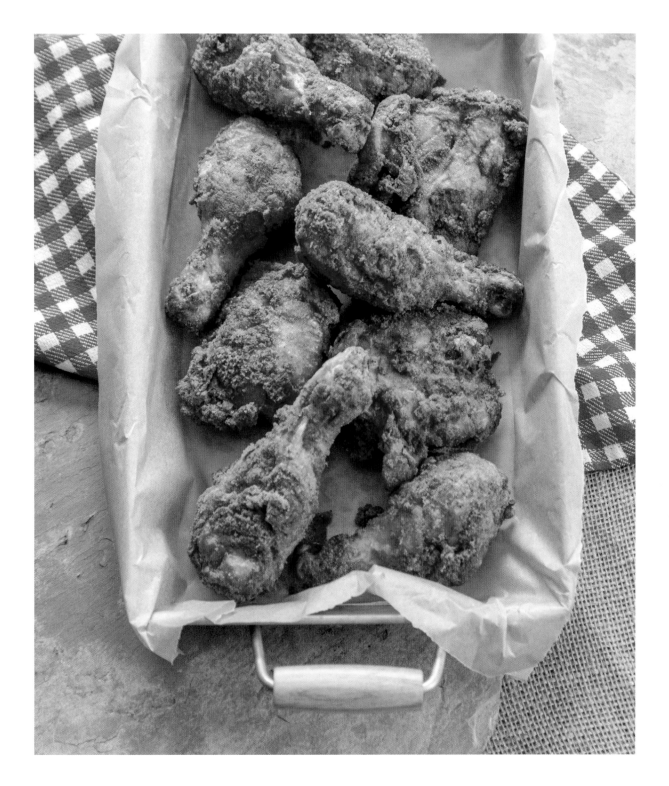

NET CARBS 2.1g				
calories	fat	protein	carbs	fiber
648	31g	87.1g	3g	0.9g

Note:

Do not use an air fryer for this recipe! The whey protein powder requires hot oil for the right results. Though it's not a traditional breading, whey powder gives breaded and fried foods a light and crispy texture, making it perfect for this fried chicken recipe.

Barbecue Pulled Pork Pizza

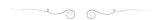

yield: 4 servings
prep time: 20 minutes
cook time: 30 minutes

The crust of this Southern-themed pizza is made with the famous keto mozzarella dough. I've found that chilling the dough before rolling it out makes it easier to work with. Don't be intimidated by making your own pizza crust; it takes a few extra steps, but it's worth it!

CRUST:

2 cups shredded mozzarella cheese

2 ounces cream cheese (¼ cup)

¾ cup finely ground blanched almond flour

1 large egg

2 teaspoons baking powder

1 teaspoon garlic powder

TOPPINGS:

½ cup Easy BBQ Sauce (page 277), plus extra for serving

1 cup shredded mozzarella cheese

1 cup shredded Slow Cooker Pulled Pork (page 158) or store-bought pulled pork

2 mini sweet peppers, sliced

1. Preheat the oven to 425°F.

2. Make the crust: Put the mozzarella and cream cheese in a large microwave-safe bowl. Microwave for 90 seconds, stirring every 30 seconds. Remove from the microwave and stir until melted and smooth.

3. Add the almond flour, egg, and baking powder to the cheese mixture and stir to combine. Microwave for 10 seconds and stir again. Using your hands, mix the ingredients until they're completely combined and a firm dough comes together. If the dough sticks to your hands, put a little olive oil on your hands and continue. Place the dough in the refrigerator for 10 minutes.

4. Remove the dough from the refrigerator and place it between two sheets of parchment paper. Use a rolling pin to roll the dough to a ¼-inch thickness in your desired shape. Remove the top sheet of parchment.

5. Leaving the crust on the bottom sheet of parchment paper, transfer it to a pizza pan or baking sheet. Use a fork to lightly prick holes throughout the crust. Par-bake the crust for 10 minutes, then remove it from the oven and use a fork to pop any bubbles that have formed. Return the crust to the oven and bake until golden brown, 5 to 8 more minutes. Leave the oven on.

6. Spread the BBQ sauce evenly over the par-baked crust. Top the sauce with the mozzarella, pulled pork, and sliced peppers. Bake the pizza for 10 minutes or until the cheese is melted. Serve with additional BBQ sauce.

NET CARBS 4.8g				
calories	fat	protein	carbs	fiber
274	19.8g	16.5g	6.6g	1.8g

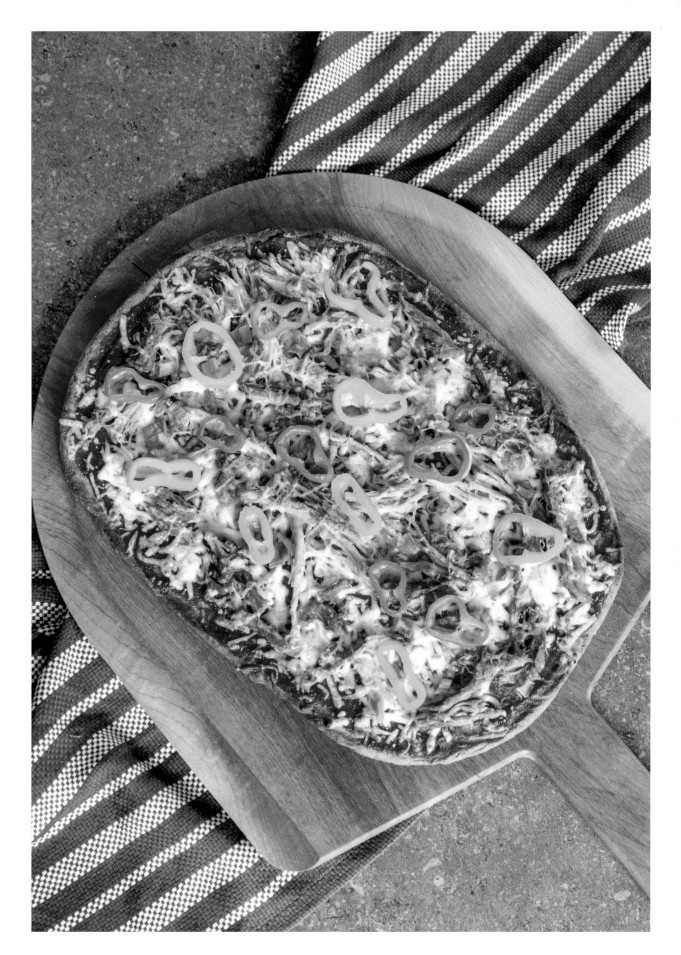

Salmon Patties

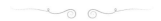

yield: 6 patties (2 per serving)

prep time: 10 minutes, plus 20 minutes to chill

cook time: 24 minutes

Growing up, salmon patties were one of my favorite foods to find left over on the stovetop when I visited my grandparents. That and potato soup! My grandma made the best salmon patties, and I'm pretty sure they had crushed crackers in them. You can eat these salmon patties without worrying about hidden carbs!

1 (14¾-ounce) can wild-caught pink salmon

1 large egg

¼ cup finely ground blanched almond flour

¼ cup grated Parmesan cheese

2 tablespoons mayonnaise

1 tablespoon finely chopped onions

1 tablespoon chopped fresh chives

1 tablespoon dried parsley

1 teaspoon freshly squeezed lemon juice

½ teaspoon ground black pepper

¼ teaspoon garlic powder

¼ teaspoon salt

High-quality oil, for frying

Sliced fresh chives, for garnish (optional)

1. Drain the salmon and put it in a large mixing bowl. If you prefer, remove any pieces of skin or bone.

2. To the bowl, add the egg, almond flour, Parmesan cheese, mayonnaise, onions, chives, parsley, lemon juice, pepper, garlic powder, and salt. Use a spoon to thoroughly combine the ingredients.

3. Shape the salmon mixture into 6 equal patties. Place the salmon patties in the refrigerator for 20 minutes. This will help them hold together better when cooked.

4. Heat enough oil to cover the bottom of a medium-sized skillet. Over medium-high heat, pan-fry the patties in two batches for 5 to 6 minutes on each side, until golden brown. Serve immediately. Garnish with more chives, if desired.

NET CARBS 2.8g				
calories	fat	protein	carbs	fiber
520	39.2g	37g	5.3g	2.5g

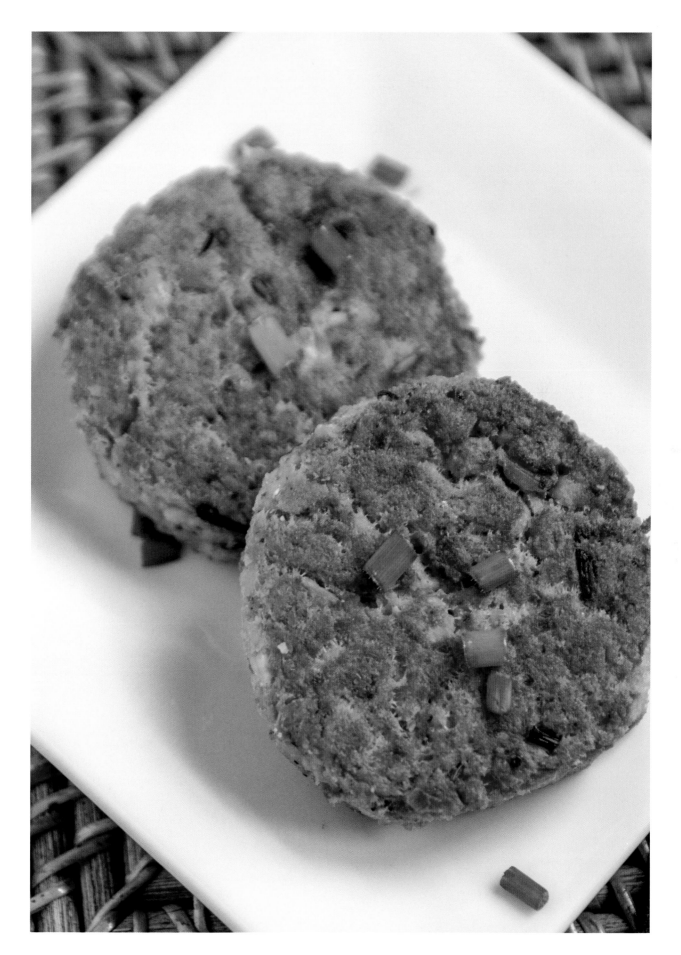

Pizza-Stuffed Peppers

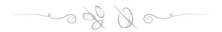

yield: 4 servings
prep time: 20 minutes
cook time: 25 minutes

My husband isn't a picky eater, but there are two foods he's always told me he won't eat: stuffed peppers and any preparation of eggplant. Well, I changed his mind with these pizza-stuffed peppers! It turns out that he's not a fan of stuffed green peppers, but any other color is fine. And you can't go wrong with a pizza-inspired filling!

1 pound Italian sausage, casings removed

1 cup marinara sauce

4 bell peppers (red, orange, yellow, or a combination)

1 cup shredded mozzarella cheese

16 slices pepperoni

Italian seasoning, for sprinkling

Grated Parmesan cheese, for garnish

1. In a medium-sized skillet over medium heat, cook the sausage until browned and no longer pink, crumbling the meat with a large spoon as it cooks. Drain the fat, if necessary. Stir in the marinara sauce and set aside.

2. Preheat the oven to 375°F. Line a sheet pan with parchment paper.

3. Cut each pepper in half lengthwise and remove the seeds. Fill the pepper halves with the sausage mixture, then top each pepper half with 2 tablespoons of the mozzarella and 2 slices of pepperoni. Sprinkle each pepper half with Italian seasoning.

4. Bake for 20 to 25 minutes, until the peppers are tender and the cheese is bubbly. Garnish with grated Parmesan.

NET CARBS 2.8g				
calories	fat	protein	carbs	fiber
287	23.7g	13.1g	5.2g	1.5g

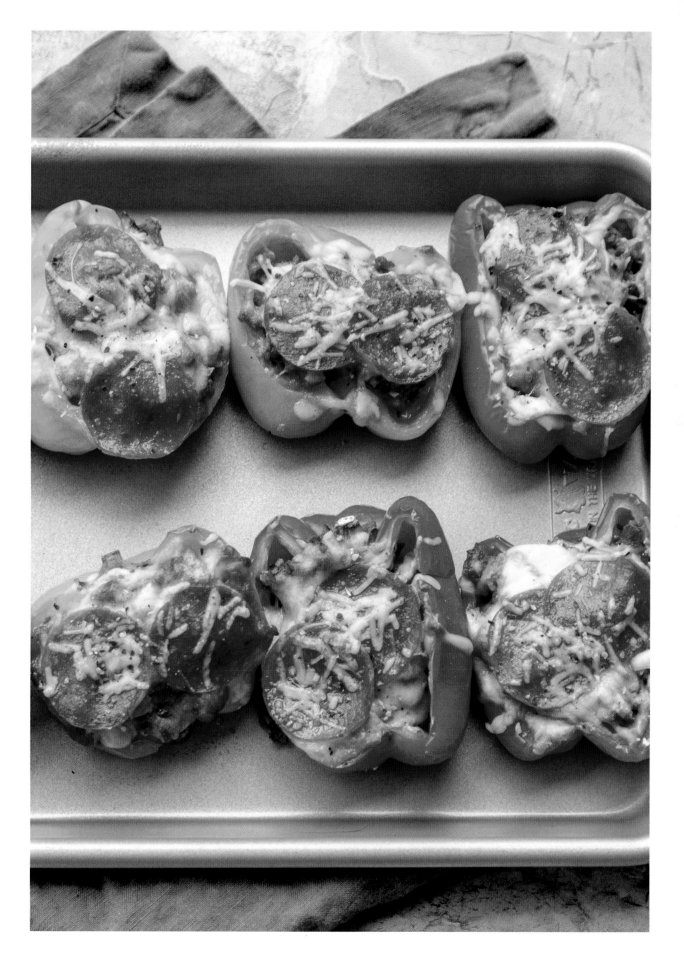

Butter Roasted Turkey

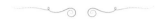

yield: 12 servings

prep time: 20 minutes

cook time: 3 hours 30 minutes

1 (12-pound) whole turkey

¾ cup (1½ sticks) unsalted butter, cut into 1-tablespoon portions

4 cups chicken broth

¼ cup finely chopped onions

¼ cup chopped fresh flat-leaf parsley

2 tablespoons seasoning salt

My husband makes this turkey every year for Thanksgiving, and it is the star of our Southern table. No dry turkey here; it's so moist and tender!

1. Preheat the oven to 350°F. Remove the neck and the packet of giblets from the turkey's cavity. Rinse the turkey and pat it dry.

2. Place the turkey breast side up in a roasting pan. Separate the skin of the breast and legs from the meat by gently sliding your fingers underneath the skin. This makes pockets into which you can place the pats of butter. Distribute the pats of butter evenly over the turkey breast and legs.

3. Combine the broth, onions, and parsley in a bowl. Pour the broth mixture over the turkey. Sprinkle the seasoning salt evenly over the turkey.

4. Insert an oven-safe meat thermometer into the lower part of the thigh, making sure that the thermometer probe does not come into contact with the bone. Loosely cover the turkey with aluminum foil. Roast the turkey for 3 to 3½ hours, basting the bird with the pan juices every 30 minutes. In the last 30 minutes of cooking, remove the foil so that the skin turns golden brown. When the turkey is done, it should have an internal temperature of 180°F in the thigh and 165°F in the breast.

5. Transfer the turkey to a carving board or platter to rest for 15 minutes before you carve it. Leftovers can be stored in an airtight container in the refrigerator for up to 4 days.

NET CARBS 0.3g				
calories	fat	protein	carbs	fiber
264	18.1g	25.9g	0.4g	0.1g

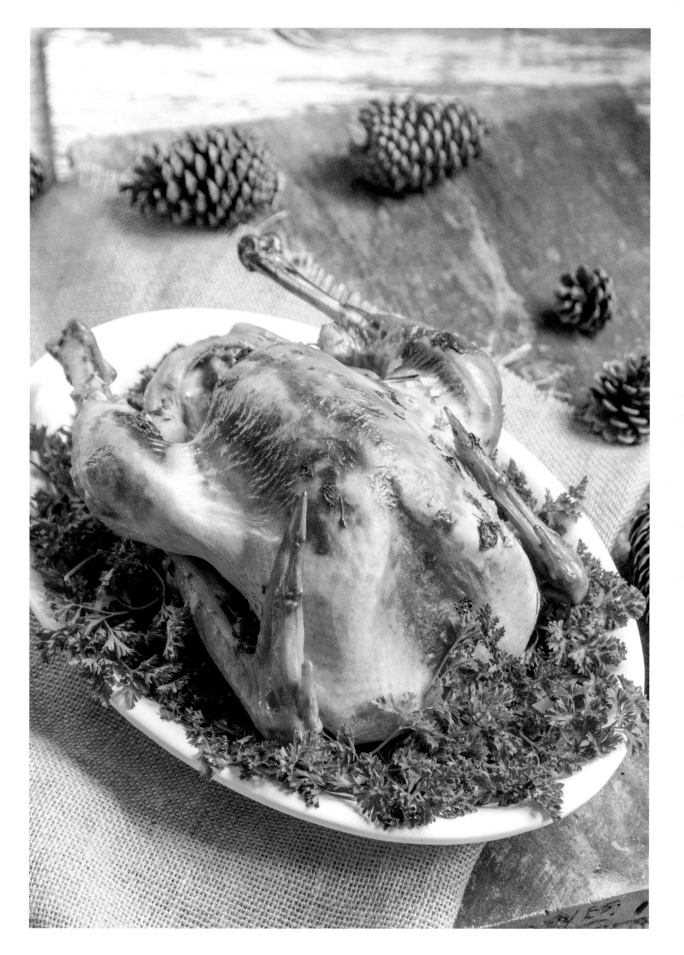

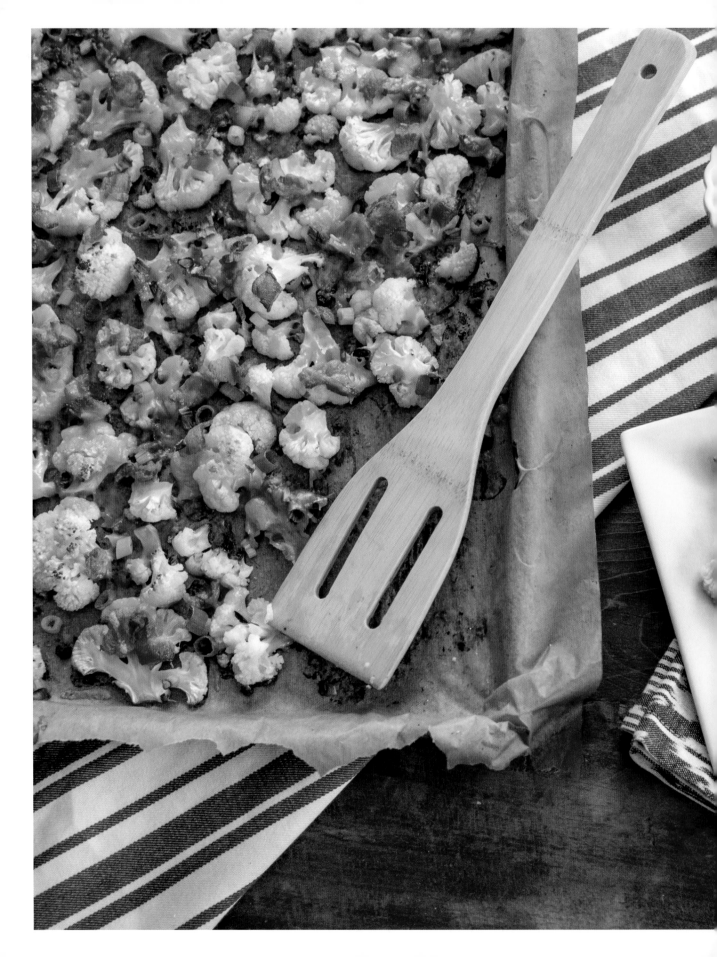

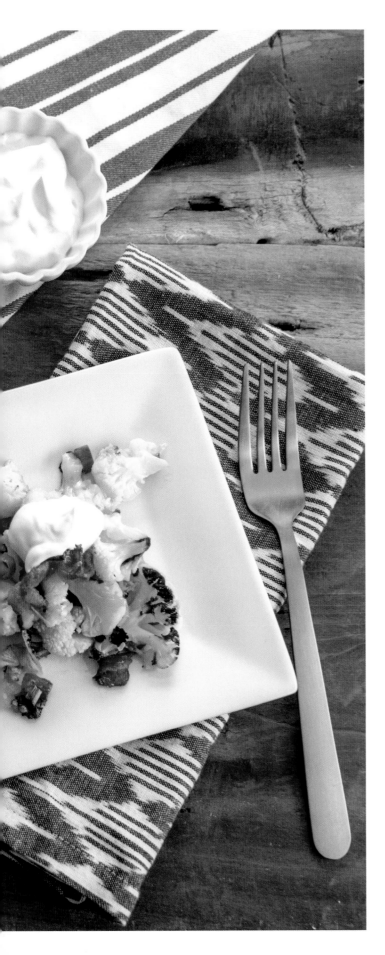

Side Dishes

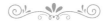

Fried Cabbage and Bacon

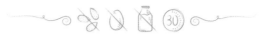

yield: 4 servings

prep time: 5 minutes

cook time: 15 minutes

I remember my mom frying cabbage; back then I never liked it. Turns out it's another one of those foods that I appreciated more as I got older. And I'm pretty sure Mom didn't put bacon in hers! Remember, bacon was a "bad-for-you" food in the 1980s.

4 slices bacon, chopped

1 medium head green cabbage, coarsely chopped

½ teaspoon salt

¾ teaspoon ground black pepper

1. In a medium-sized skillet over medium heat, cook the bacon until crispy. Use a slotted spoon to remove the bacon and set it aside.

2. Put the cabbage in the skillet with the bacon drippings and cook, stirring frequently, for about 10 minutes, until tender. Return the bacon to the pan, add the salt and pepper, and continue cooking for 5 more minutes. Serve immediately.

NET CARBS 5g				
calories	fat	protein	carbs	fiber
86	4.7g	5g	8.8g	3.9g

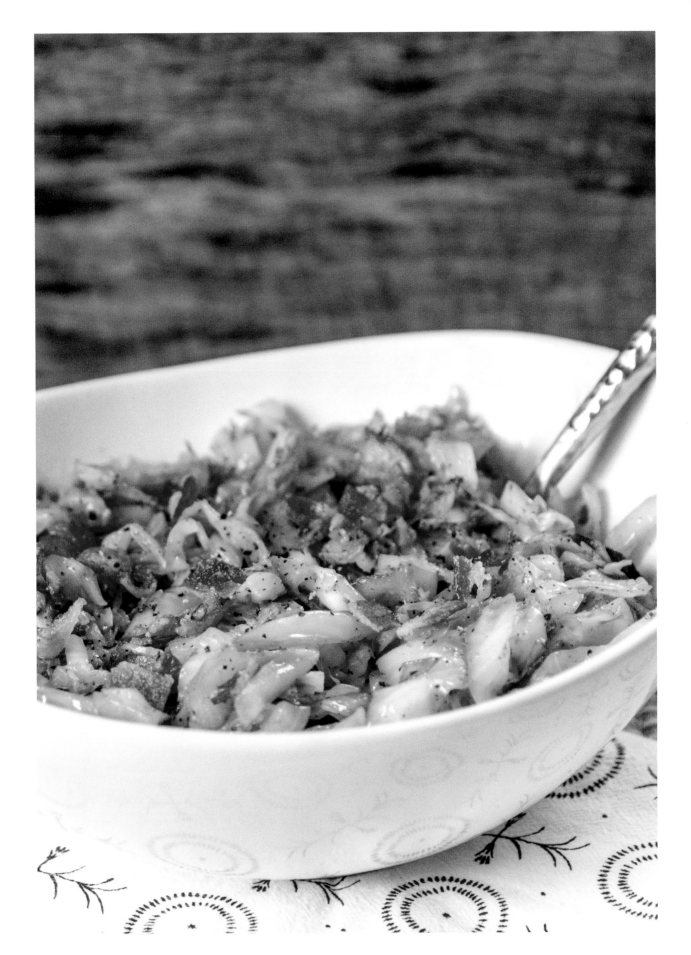

Green Bean Bacon Bundles

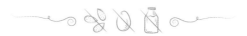

yield: 4 servings

prep time: 15 minutes

cook time: 25 minutes

Green beans have always been one of my favorite vegetables. My grandma would cook green beans fresh from the garden with ham, and she would let them simmer all day. I still love them prepared that way, but these little bundles are great, too, and they don't take much time to make.

12 ounces fresh green beans (about 2 cups), trimmed

2 tablespoons avocado oil

8 slices bacon, cut in half crosswise

½ teaspoon salt

¼ teaspoon ground black pepper

1. Preheat the oven to 400°F. Line a sheet pan with parchment paper.

2. Toss the green beans in the oil.

3. Using the bacon slices, wrap the green beans into bundles of 4 or 5 beans each. The number per bundle will depend on the length of the bacon and thickness of the beans. Place each bundle on the prepared pan with the seam of the bacon facedown. Sprinkle evenly with the salt and pepper.

4. Bake for 25 minutes or until the bacon reaches the desired crispness and the green beans are tender.

NET CARBS 2.1g				
calories	fat	protein	carbs	fiber
186	16.1g	7.9g	3.5g	1.4g

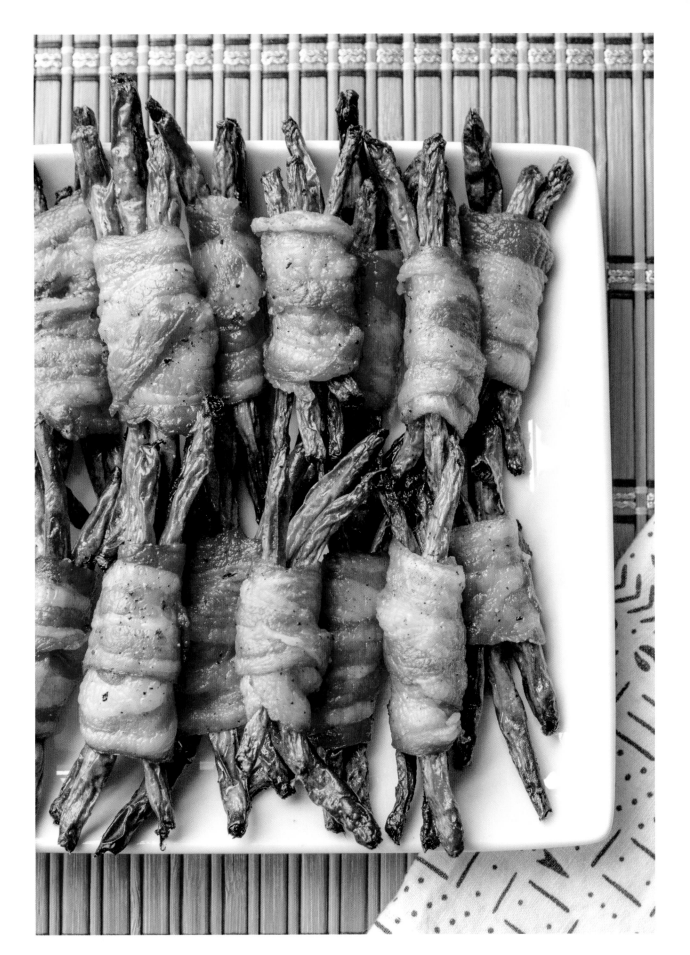

Loaded Roasted Cauliflower

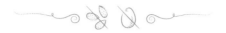

yield: 4 servings
prep time: 10 minutes
cook time: 30 minutes

When I shared this recipe on Instagram, it was an instant hit! It also went straight to the top of my family's list of favorite recipes. I know you're thinking it sounds the same as loaded caulimash or casserole, but it's not. Roasting the cauliflower makes the flavor so much better. I haven't had real cheese fries from a restaurant in a long time, but this dish comes very close to that flavor! It's delicious served with sour cream or Ranch Dressing (page 274).

1 medium head cauliflower

2 tablespoons avocado oil

Salt

2 slices bacon, chopped

2 green onions, sliced

1 cup shredded sharp cheddar cheese

1. Preheat the oven to 400°F. Line a sheet pan with parchment paper.

2. Core the cauliflower and cut the florets into bite-sized pieces. Toss the cauliflower with the oil, then spread it on the lined sheet pan and sprinkle lightly with salt. Top the cauliflower evenly with the bacon and green onions.

3. Bake for 25 minutes, then remove from the oven and top with the cheese. Bake for 2 to 4 more minutes, until the cheese is melted.

NET CARBS 5.5g				
calories	fat	protein	carbs	fiber
242	19.1g	11.1g	8.5g	3g

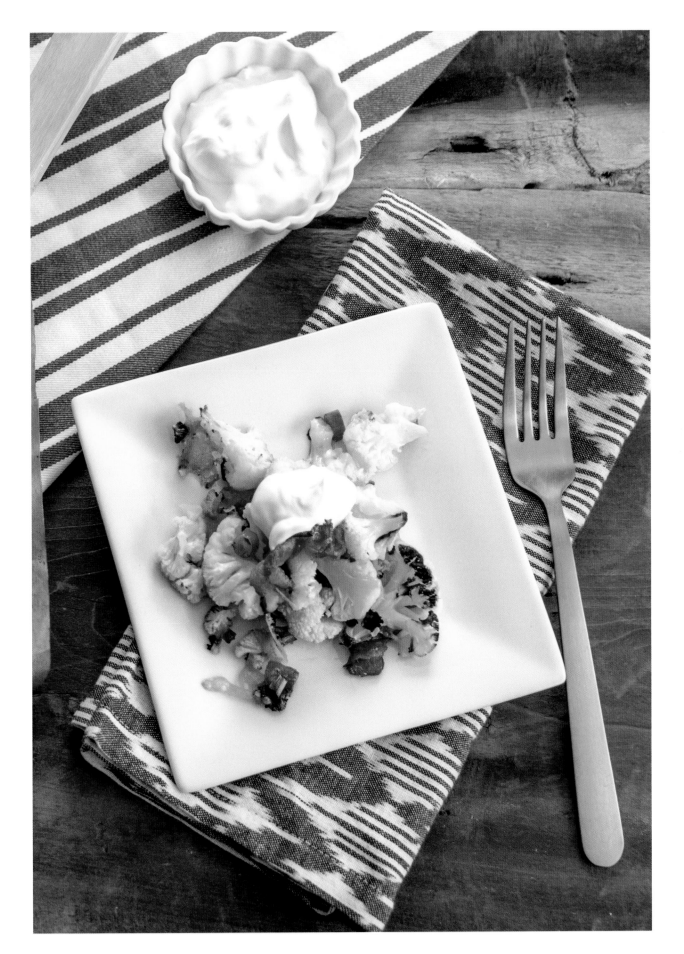

Hash Brown Casserole

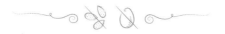

yield: 6 servings
prep time: 5 minutes
cook time: 38 minutes

Hash brown casserole has long been a favorite to take to church potlucks in the South. But how do you make hash brown casserole without potatoes? You guessed it: cauliflower! The hash brown casserole I ate when I was growing up was topped with cornflakes. For a little added crunch, I top mine with a mixture of Parmesan cheese and pork rinds. You can leave off the topping if you prefer.

2 tablespoons salted butter

¼ cup chopped onions

½ cup heavy whipping cream

½ teaspoon salt

½ teaspoon ground black pepper

1 (12-ounce) bag frozen riced cauliflower

1½ cups shredded cheddar cheese

TOPPING (optional):

¾ cup crushed pork rinds

¼ cup grated Parmesan cheese

1. Preheat the oven to 350°F. Grease an 11 by 8-inch or similar-sized oval baking dish.

2. Melt the butter in a medium-sized skillet over medium heat. Sauté the onions in the butter until tender and translucent. Reduce the heat to low and stir in the cream, salt, and pepper. Simmer for 2 minutes, then stir in the cauliflower and cheddar cheese.

3. Transfer the mixture to the prepared baking dish. Bake the casserole for 25 minutes, or until browned and bubbly around the edges.

4. While the casserole is baking, make the topping, if using: Mix together the pork rinds and Parmesan cheese. Sprinkle the topping evenly over the casserole and bake for 5 more minutes, or until the topping is lightly browned.

5. Leftovers can be stored in an airtight container in the refrigerator for up to 3 days.

NET CARBS 3.3g				
calories	fat	protein	carbs	fiber
278	22.3g	13.1g	4.8g	1.5g

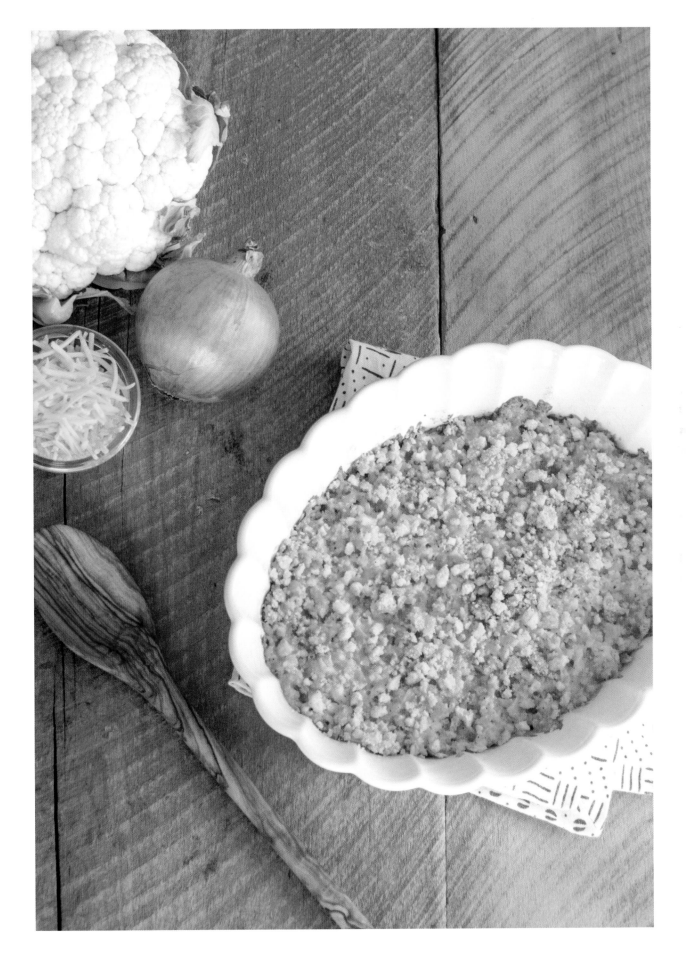

Easy Cheesy Caulirice

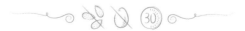

yield: 4 servings

prep time: 5 minutes

cook time: 20 minutes

I make this comforting side dish at least once a week! It's a favorite of ours and goes with everything. It's what we consider a rich and creamy substitute for mac and cheese. You won't believe how easy it is to make!

2 tablespoons salted butter

1 (12-ounce) bag frozen riced cauliflower

½ cup shredded cheddar cheese

2 tablespoons heavy whipping cream

Salt and ground black pepper

1. Melt the butter in a medium-sized skillet over medium heat.

2. Put the cauliflower in the skillet and cook, stirring occasionally, until tender, about 15 minutes.

3. Turn off the heat. Add the cheese and cream to the skillet and stir until the cheese is completely melted and the ingredients are fully combined.

4. Season to taste with salt and pepper. Serve immediately.

Variation:

Basic Caulirice. Omit the cheese and cream. Complete Steps 1 and 2 as written, then season the caulirice to taste with salt and pepper and serve.

NET CARBS 2.7g				
calories	fat	protein	carbs	fiber
156	13.5g	5.1g	4.6g	2g

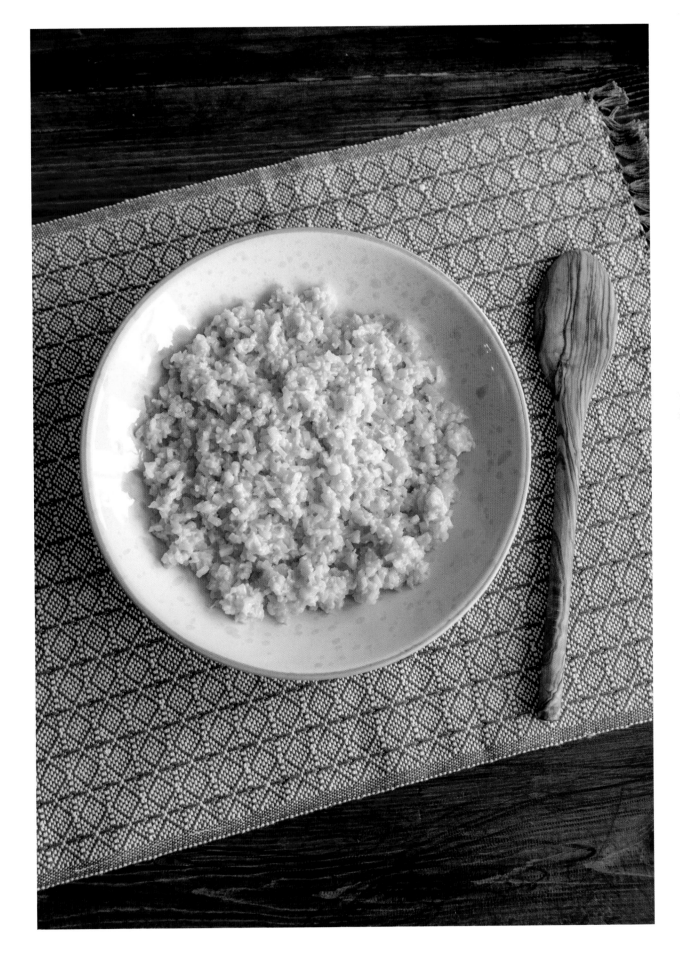

Roasted Spaghetti Squash

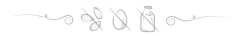

yield: 8 servings
prep time: 10 minutes
cook time: 52 minutes

This is another versatile side dish. You can stuff the squash halves with a filling, or you can serve the squash threads like spaghetti topped with marinara or Alfredo sauce. Really, the possible uses for spaghetti squash are endless!

1 spaghetti squash (about 4 pounds)

2 tablespoons avocado oil

Salt and ground black pepper

1. Preheat the oven to 400°F. Line a sheet pan with parchment paper.

2. Use a knife to pierce holes down both sides of the squash. Microwave the squash on high power for 7 minutes. Carefully remove using oven mitts; the squash will be hot.

3. Slice the squash in half lengthwise. Use a spoon to scoop out the seeds.

4. Drizzle the squash halves with the oil and sprinkle evenly with salt and pepper. Place cut side down on the lined sheet pan and roast in the oven for 45 minutes, until the skin is softened.

5. Allow the squash to cool, then use a fork to shred it. Leftovers can be stored in an airtight container in the refrigerator for up to 5 days.

NET CARBS 3.9g				
calories	fat	protein	carbs	fiber
46	0.3g	0.5g	5g	1.1g

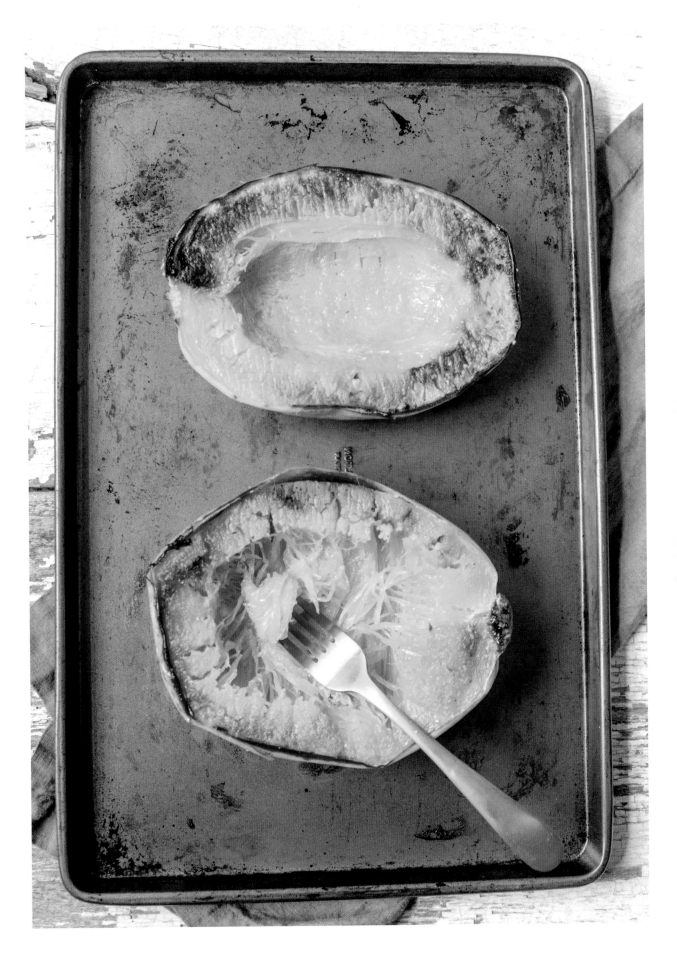

Turnip Fries with Dipping Sauce

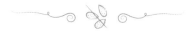

yield: 6 servings
prep time: 15 minutes
cook time: 30 minutes

I don't know what took me so long to discover turnips as a fit for our ketogenic lifestyle! Sometimes we really miss french fries, and these are a great substitute. Though they don't quite duplicate the crispness of a french fry, the texture is similar, and they are very satisfying, especially when served with my tangy homemade dipping sauce. If you don't feel like making the dipping sauce, sugar-free ketchup is a nice option, too!

FRIES:

4 medium turnips

2 tablespoons avocado oil

½ cup grated Parmesan cheese

1 teaspoon paprika

½ teaspoon chili powder

½ teaspoon garlic powder

DIPPING SAUCE:

½ cup mayonnaise

¼ cup sugar-free ketchup

2 tablespoons dill relish

1½ teaspoons white vinegar

¼ teaspoon ground black pepper

⅛ teaspoon salt

1. Preheat the oven to 425°F. Line a sheet pan with parchment paper.

2. Make the fries: Peel the turnips and cut them into 3 by ¼-inch sticks. In a large bowl, toss the fries in the oil to coat.

3. Put the Parmesan cheese, paprika, chili powder, and garlic powder in a separate bowl and stir to combine. Add the oiled fries to the seasoning mixture and toss to coat evenly. Spread the fries on the prepared pan.

4. Bake for 30 minutes or until the fries are brown and crisp around the edges, turning them halfway through for even browning.

5. Meanwhile, make the dipping sauce: Place all the sauce ingredients in a small bowl and stir to combine.

6. When the fries are done, remove from the oven and serve immediately with the dipping sauce.

Note:
If you find turnips with the greens on them, don't discard the greens. Braise them in bacon drippings in a cast-iron skillet for a tasty Southern side dish known simply as "greens."

NET CARBS 4.8g				
calories	fat	protein	carbs	fiber
224	21g	2.7g	6.5g	1.7g

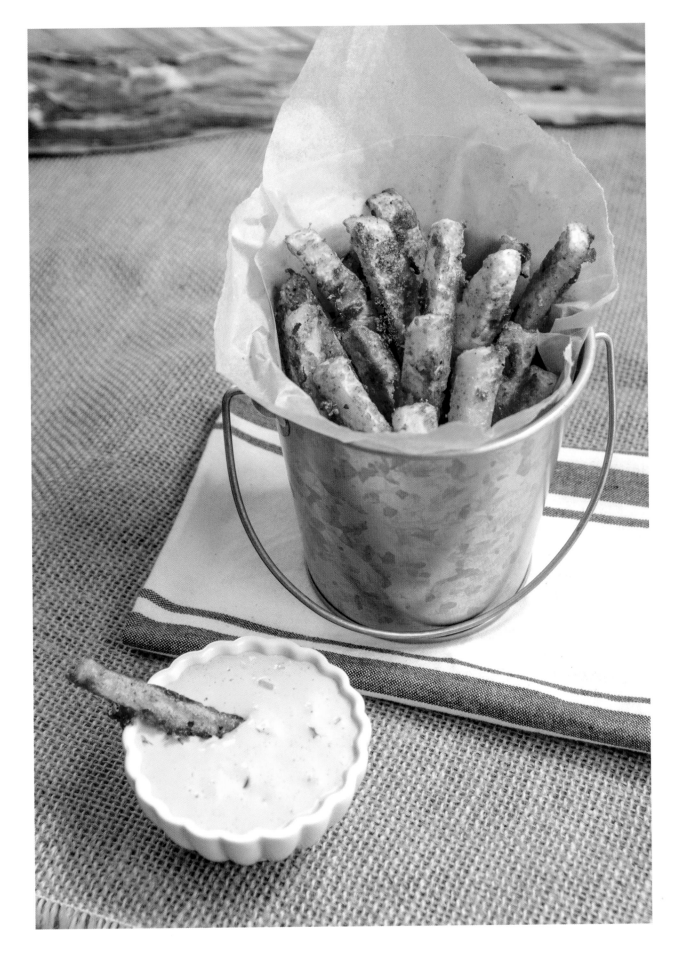

Sausage Cornbread Dressing

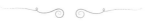

yield: 8 servings

prep time: 20 minutes (not including time to make cornbread)

cook time: 30 minutes

There's so much to say about this dish! I'll start with the fact that I call it dressing instead of stuffing. I know, I know; there's much debate on that! Where I'm from, we call it dressing; therefore it is and always will be dressing. I've been making this for the last couple of years for Thanksgiving dinner, and I finally nailed down the proper measurements for you. I originally made it by taste, and, well, you can't put that in a cookbook. I hope you enjoy finally being able to have a low-carb dressing with your turkey during the holidays!

1 recipe Skillet Cornbread (page 74), cooled

1 pound bulk breakfast sausage

½ cup diced onions

2 ribs celery, diced

2 large eggs

2 tablespoons salted butter, melted but not hot

2 teaspoons ground dried sage

¼ teaspoon salt

¼ teaspoon ground black pepper

1½ cups vegetable broth

1. Preheat the oven to 350°F. Grease an 8 by 11-inch baking dish.

2. In a large mixing bowl, crumble the cornbread into bite-sized pieces and set aside.

3. In a medium-sized skillet over medium heat, cook the sausage with the onions and celery, crumbling the meat with a large spoon as it cooks, until the sausage is browned and the vegetables are tender. Drain and set aside.

4. In a small bowl, whisk together the eggs and melted butter. Stir in the sage, salt, and pepper. Pour the egg mixture over the cornbread and stir gently.

5. Add the sausage mixture to the cornbread and stir gently. Pour in the broth and stir gently until well combined.

6. Spread the dressing evenly in the prepared baking dish and bake for 30 minutes or until the top is browned. Allow to cool for 10 minutes before serving. Leftovers can be stored in an airtight container in the refrigerator for up to 5 days.

NET CARBS 4g				
calories	fat	protein	carbs	fiber
455	40.9g	9.8g	5g	3g

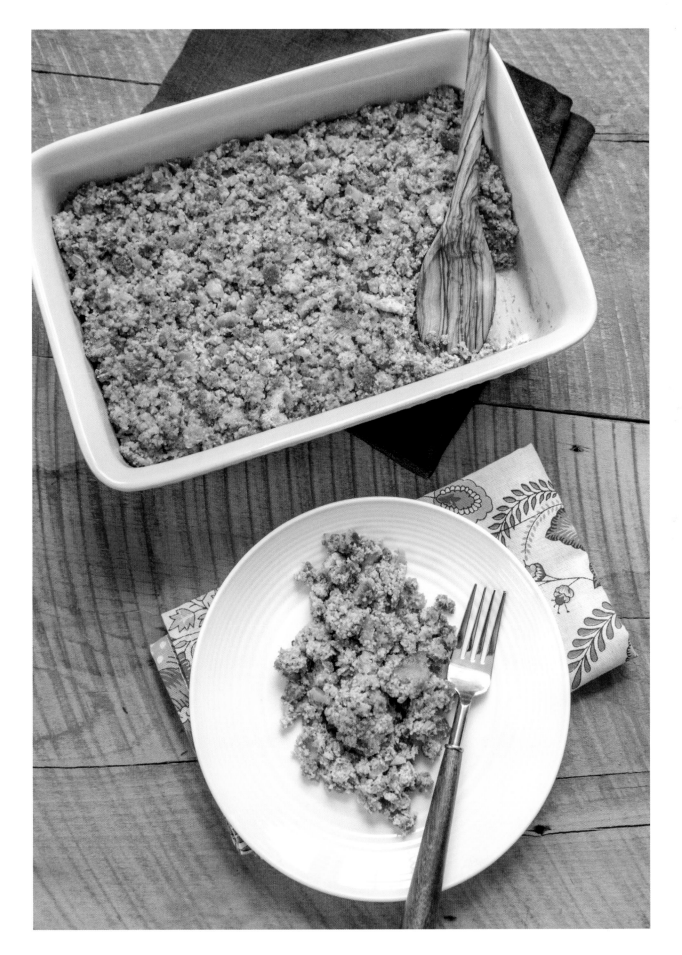

Easy Caulimash

yield: 4 servings

prep time: 5 minutes

cook time: 10 minutes

Here's a super easy keto substitute for mashed potatoes. A food processor or high-powered blender isn't absolutely necessary, but it makes a difference in the texture. Follow this recipe for smooth and creamy mash. Don't skip the step of draining the excess liquid; you don't want watery caulimash!

1 (12-ounce) bag frozen cauliflower florets

3 tablespoons salted butter, plus extra for garnish if desired

2 tablespoons heavy whipping cream

Salt and ground black pepper

1. Cook the cauliflower according to the package directions. Drain the excess liquid.

2. Place the cauliflower in a food processor or high-powered blender. Add the butter and cream and pulse until the mixture is smooth and creamy. Season to taste with salt and pepper.

3. Put the caulimash in a serving bowl and garnish with more butter, if desired.

Note:

You also can use an immersion blender to mash the cauliflower in Step 2.

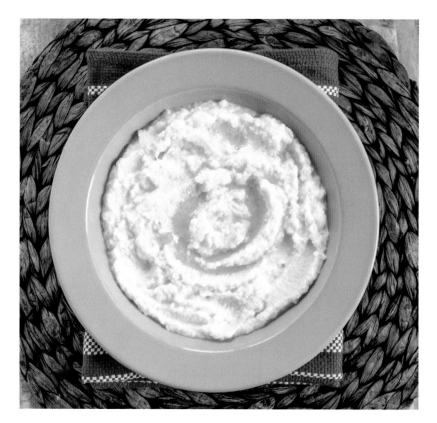

NET CARBS 4.9g				
calories	fat	protein	carbs	fiber
151	12g	4.2g	9.5g	4.6g

Parmesan Asparagus

yield: 4 servings

prep time: 5 minutes

cook time: 30 minutes

Asparagus is a vegetable that I frequently order at restaurants, but really, I prefer my way of making it at home. This is a great side dish to pair with the Reverse Sear Garlic Rosemary Rib-Eye Steaks (page 176).

1 pound asparagus spears

2 tablespoons extra-virgin olive oil

Salt

¾ cup shredded or grated Parmesan cheese

1. Preheat the oven to 425°F. Line a sheet pan with parchment paper.

2. Trim the tough ends off the asparagus spears. Toss the asparagus in the oil and spread evenly on the lined sheet pan. Sprinkle lightly with salt.

3. Bake for 25 minutes, or until the asparagus is tender. Remove from the oven and sprinkle the Parmesan cheese evenly over the asparagus. Return to the oven for 5 more minutes, or until the cheese starts to brown and crisp. Serve immediately.

Note:

The cooking time can vary according to the thickness of the asparagus you choose. If the spears are quite thick, you might need to cook them longer than 25 minutes before topping with the cheese.

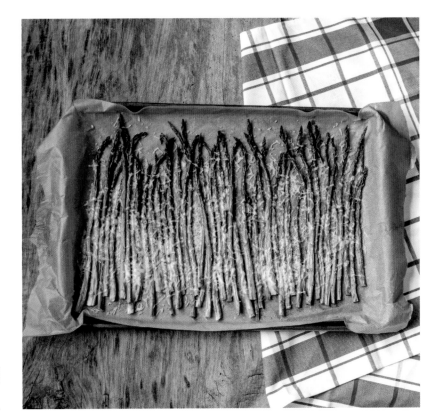

NET CARBS 2.4g				
calories	fat	protein	carbs	fiber
126	9.8g	6.5g	4.8g	2.4g

Garlic Butter Roasted Radishes

yield: 4 servings

prep time: 10 minutes

cook time: 25 minutes

When cooked this way, radishes remind me of the little potatoes my papa used to grow in his garden. The taste isn't exactly like a potato, but the texture is right, and when you pair the radishes with butter and garlic, you can't go wrong!

1 pound radishes

3 tablespoons salted butter, melted (see Note)

2 cloves garlic, minced

Salt

Ground black pepper

1. Preheat the oven to 425°F. Line a sheet pan with parchment paper.

2. Trim the ends off the radishes and cut them in half. Coat the radishes evenly in the melted butter and garlic, then spread them on the lined sheet pan. Generously sprinkle with salt.

3. Bake for 25 minutes or until slightly golden brown, turning the radishes halfway through the baking time. Garnish with freshly ground black pepper and serve.

Note:

Using a good-quality grass-fed butter really makes a difference in this recipe.

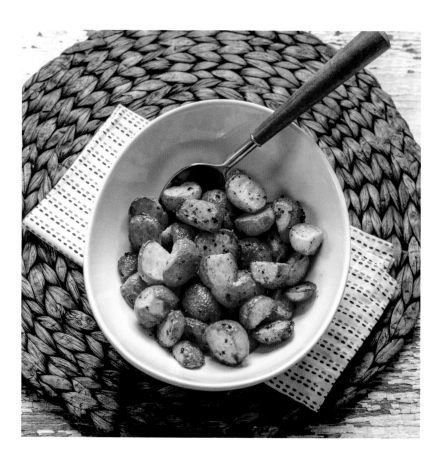

NET CARBS 2.5g				
calories	fat	protein	carbs	fiber
71	5.9g	0.9g	4.4g	1.8g

Bacon Roasted Cabbage Steaks

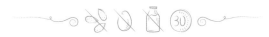

yield: 4 servings
prep time: 10 minutes
cook time: 20 minutes

This delicious side dish is simple enough for a weeknight and fancy enough to serve to guests.

1 medium head green or red cabbage, or a combination

2 tablespoons avocado oil

4 slices bacon, chopped

Salt and ground black pepper

1. Preheat the oven to 400°F. Line a sheet pan with parchment paper.

2. Cut the base off the cabbage and set the flat end on a cutting board. Cut the cabbage into 1-inch slices and arrange them on the lined sheet pan.

3. Drizzle the oil over the cabbage slices. Top the cabbage evenly with the bacon, then season with a couple of pinches each of salt and pepper.

4. Bake for 20 minutes, until the edges of the cabbage are caramelized and the bacon is done. Serve immediately.

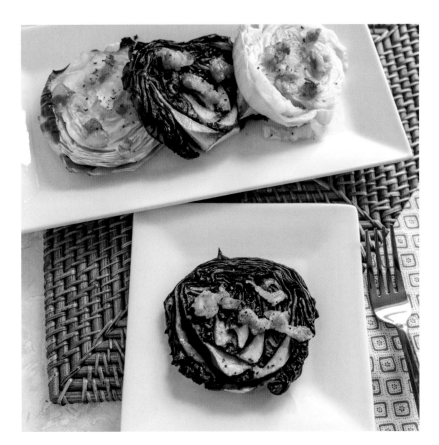

NET CARBS 4.8g				
calories	fat	protein	carbs	fiber
146	11.7g	5g	8.6g	3.8g

Old-Fashioned Green Beans

yield: 4 servings
prep time: 10 minutes
cook time: 1 hour 30 minutes

I have fond childhood memories of snapping beans on the porch with my grandma and mom. At the time, though, I had no idea how special those moments were. For that reason, I had to include a recipe for country-style slow-cooked green beans in this cookbook. This recipe takes some time but is worth the extra effort for the flavor and the delicious juices—called pot liquor—that are left over, which are great for sopping up with a biscuit. (A keto biscuit, of course!) I love the meltingly soft and tender texture of these beans, too.

1 pound fresh green beans

1½ cups vegetable broth

4 slices bacon, chopped

1 tablespoon dried minced onions, or ¼ cup chopped raw onions

½ teaspoon ground black pepper

½ teaspoon garlic powder

1 tablespoon salted butter

Salt

1. Snap the ends off the green beans and break them in half or in thirds. Place the beans in a medium-sized saucepan and add the broth, bacon, onions, pepper, and garlic powder.

2. Bring the bean mixture to a boil over medium-high heat. Continue to boil for 10 minutes, then reduce the heat to low. Cover the pot and simmer for 1 hour 20 minutes or until the beans have cooked down and the juices have reduced but aren't completely gone.

3. Stir in the butter and season to taste with salt before serving.

Note:
Ham hock, fatback, or another cut of pork can be used in place of the bacon.

NET CARBS 6.1g				
calories	fat	protein	carbs	fiber
123	5.9g	6.1g	9.4g	3.3g

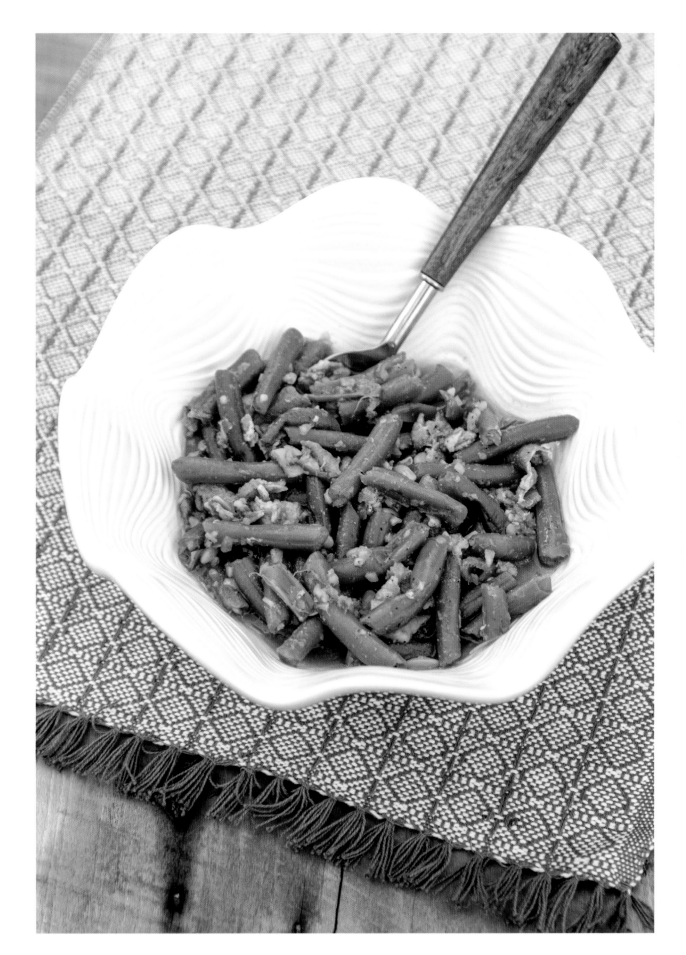

Blistered Okra

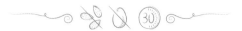

yield: 4 servings

prep time: 10 minutes

cook time: 10 minutes

Okra is a popular Southern vegetable that is often coated with flour and fried. Here's a different way to cook it that is quicker and tastier! Blistering is a high-heat cooking technique that gives vegetables a smoky flavor.

12 ounces okra

2 tablespoons salted butter

1 teaspoon Creole Seasoning (page 270) (optional)

Salt and ground black pepper

1. Slice the okra in half lengthwise.

2. Heat a 12-inch cast-iron skillet or other heavy skillet over medium-high heat. Melt the butter in the skillet.

3. Put the okra in the skillet cut side down and sear for 2 minutes. Flip the okra and cook for 2 to 3 minutes more, until blistered and charred on the edges.

4. Sprinkle on the Creole seasoning, if using, then season to taste with salt and pepper and toss to coat. Serve immediately.

NET CARBS 3.6g				
calories	fat	protein	carbs	fiber
79	5.9g	1.7g	6.3g	2.7g

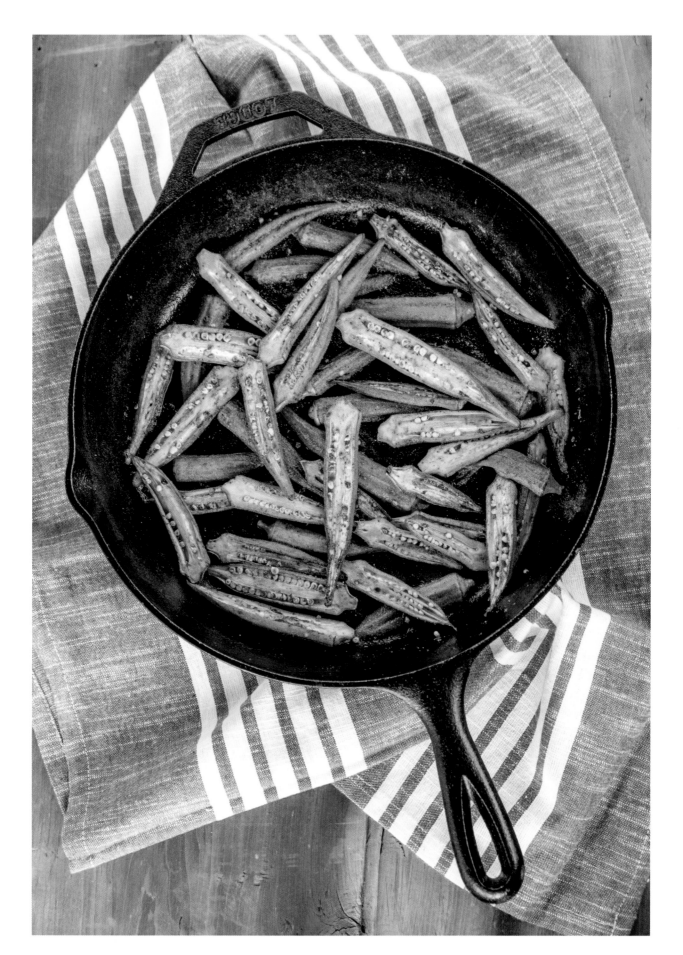

Fried Green Tomatoes

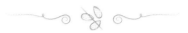

yield: 4 servings

prep time: 15 minutes

cook time: 20 minutes

3 medium-sized green tomatoes

High-quality oil, for frying

½ cup coconut flour

½ cup grated Parmesan cheese

¼ teaspoon salt

¼ teaspoon ground black pepper

1 large egg

2 tablespoons heavy whipping cream

Fried green tomatoes are a classic Southern side dish. They have a tart flavor and are so addictive—the more you eat, the more you want!

1. Cut the tomatoes into ¼-inch slices.

2. Heat ½ inch of oil in a medium-sized heavy skillet over medium heat.

3. In a shallow dish, stir together the coconut flour, Parmesan cheese, salt, and pepper. In another shallow dish, whisk together the egg and cream.

4. Dip the tomato slices into the egg mixture, allowing the excess to drip back into the dish. Then dredge the tomatoes in the flour mixture, coating both sides.

5. Working in small batches, fry the tomatoes for 2 to 3 minutes on each side, until golden brown. Add more oil as needed between batches.

6. Sprinkle lightly with more salt and serve immediately.

Note:

For extra flavor, use bacon grease instead of oil for frying.

NET CARBS 5.9g				
calories	fat	protein	carbs	fiber
152	8.4g	8.1g	9.7g	3.8g

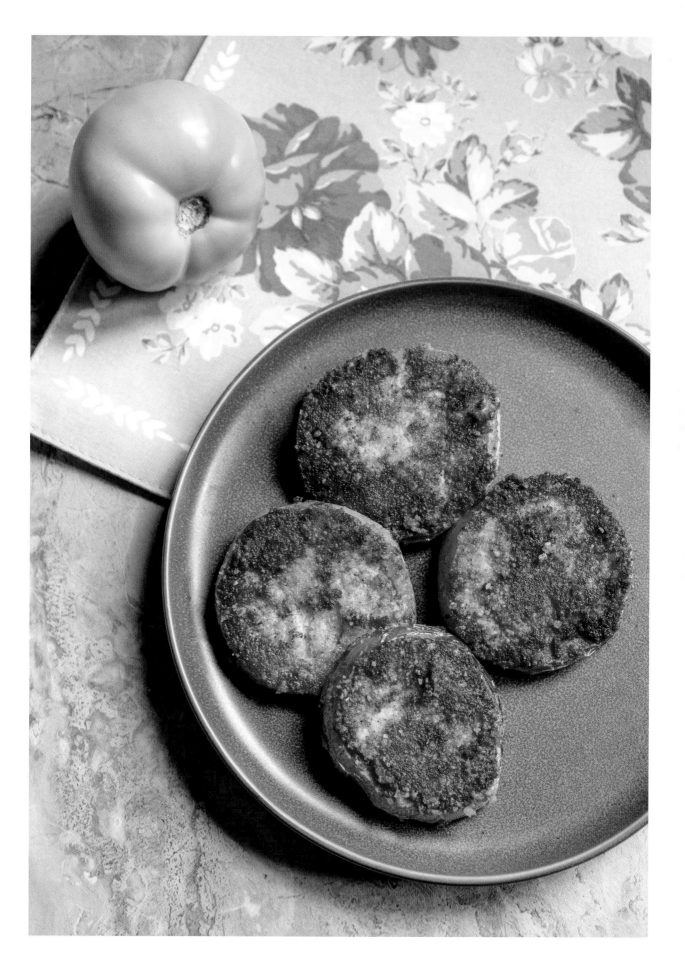

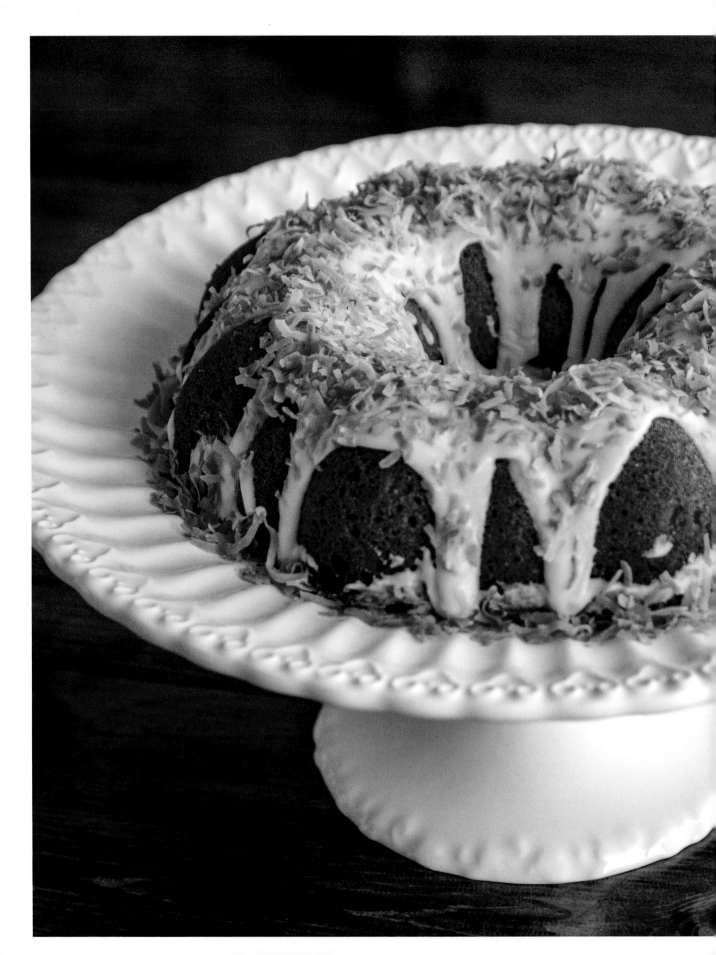

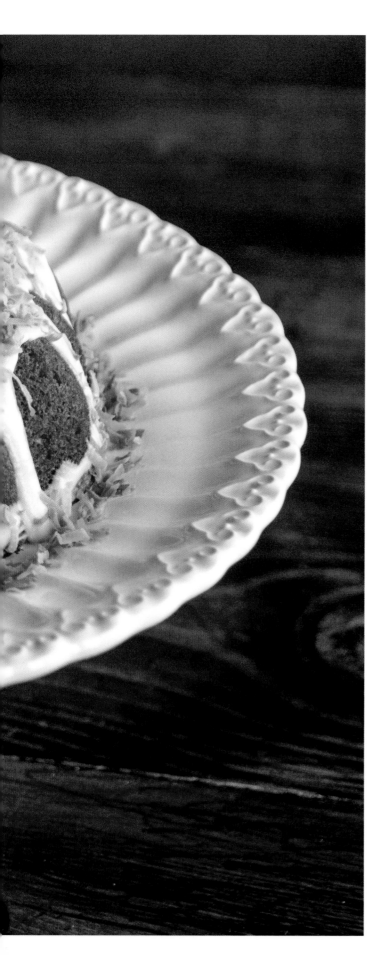

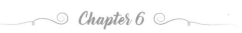
Desserts

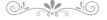

Keto Cheesecake
with Pecan Almond Crust

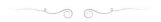

yield: 16 servings

*prep time: 20 minutes, plus
8 hours to chill*

cook time: 1 hour 45 minutes

Cheesecake is not a Southern dessert, but it is beloved by many Southerners, including my husband. Because it is his favorite dessert and often serves as his birthday cake, it is one of the first keto dessert recipes I perfected for our family. I hope you enjoy it as much as we do! Most people can't tell the difference between this and regular cheesecake. I like to serve it with Whipped Cream (page 254) and fresh berries.

CRUST:

1 cup finely ground blanched almond flour

1 cup raw pecan halves, finely crushed

½ cup granular erythritol

¼ cup (½ stick) salted butter, cubed

FILLING:

5 (8-ounce) packages cream cheese, softened

1½ cups confectioners'-style erythritol

4 large eggs

1 cup sour cream

1 tablespoon freshly squeezed lemon juice

1 teaspoon vanilla extract

To make the crust:

1. Preheat the oven to 375°F. Grease the bottom and side of a 9- or 10-inch springform pan with butter, or line it with parchment paper cut to fit the bottom of the pan and grease the sides.

2. Place all the crust ingredients in a mixing bowl and mix with a fork until well combined. The mixture will be crumbly. Press the crust mixture into the prepared pan.

3. Par-bake the crust for 12 to 15 minutes, until brown around the edges.

4. Remove the crust from the oven and turn the oven temperature down to 325°F. Let the crust cool completely, then make the filling.

To make the filling:

1. Using a hand mixer, beat the cream cheese on medium speed until fluffy.

2. With the mixer still on medium speed, gradually blend in the erythritol.

3. Blend in the eggs one at a time, scraping down the bowl after each addition.

4. Beat in the sour cream, then add the lemon juice and vanilla extract. At this point, the batter will be very thick and creamy.

NET CARBS 2.3g				
calories	fat	protein	carbs	fiber
315	28.1g	8.7g	3.6g	1.3g

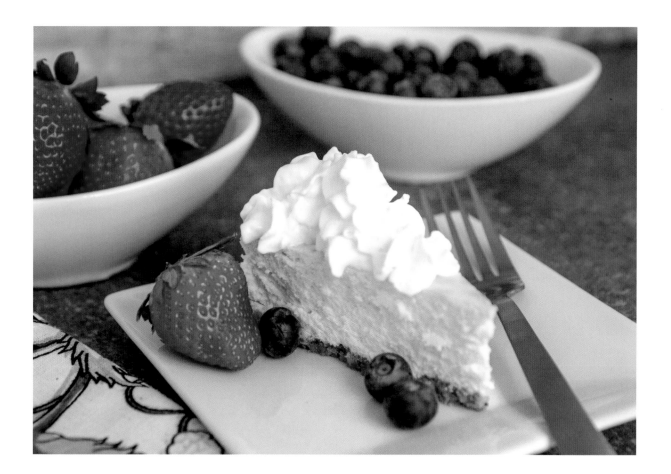

SPECIAL EQUIPMENT:

9- or 10-inch springform pan

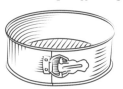

To bake the cheesecake:

1. Wrap the bottom of the cooled springform pan in aluminum foil (this will protect the cake when it sits in the water bath).

2. Pour the filling over the cooled crust, then set the springform pan inside a roasting pan.

3. Pour hot water into the roasting pan so that it comes halfway up the side of the springform pan.

4. Bake the cheesecake for 1 hour 30 minutes or until the center is firm and the top is slightly browned.

5. Remove the springform pan from the water bath. Let the cheesecake cool completely, then refrigerate for at least 8 hours or overnight.

6. Before serving, run a knife around the rim of the pan to loosen the cake, then release the side of the pan. Leftovers can be stored in an airtight container in the refrigerator for up to 5 days.

Peanut Butter
Chocolate Chip Cookie Bars

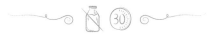

yield: 12 bars (1 per serving)
prep time: 10 minutes
cook time: 16 minutes

Southerners have long enjoyed peanuts: colonists in Virginia enjoyed savory peanut soup made with hand-ground peanuts. When peanut butter came along, dessert recipes using it proliferated—think peanut butter fudge. I love all those peanut butter treats, but I've got to say that I love peanut butter even more when it's paired with chocolate. It's one of my all-time favorite combinations! These amazing peanut butter chocolate chip bars will have you wondering how it's possible that they don't contain any type of flour.

1 cup natural peanut butter (crunchy or smooth)

2 large eggs

½ cup sugar-free chocolate chips

½ cup granular erythritol

1 teaspoon baking powder

½ teaspoon vanilla extract

5 drops liquid stevia

1. Preheat the oven to 375°F. Grease an 8-inch square baking pan.

2. Put all the ingredients in a mixing bowl. Using a wooden spoon, stir until well combined. Spread the mixture evenly in the prepared pan.

3. Bake for 14 to 16 minutes, until the edges are brown and the center is set. Watch closely and be careful not to overbake; begin checking at 14 minutes because the cookie can burn easily.

4. Allow to cool completely in the pan before cutting into 12 bars. (They will firm up as they cool.) Leftovers can be stored in an airtight container for up to a week.

Note:
You can substitute natural almond butter for the peanut butter.

NET CARBS 4.4g				
calories	fat	protein	carbs	fiber
146	12.3g	6.3g	7.1g	2.8g

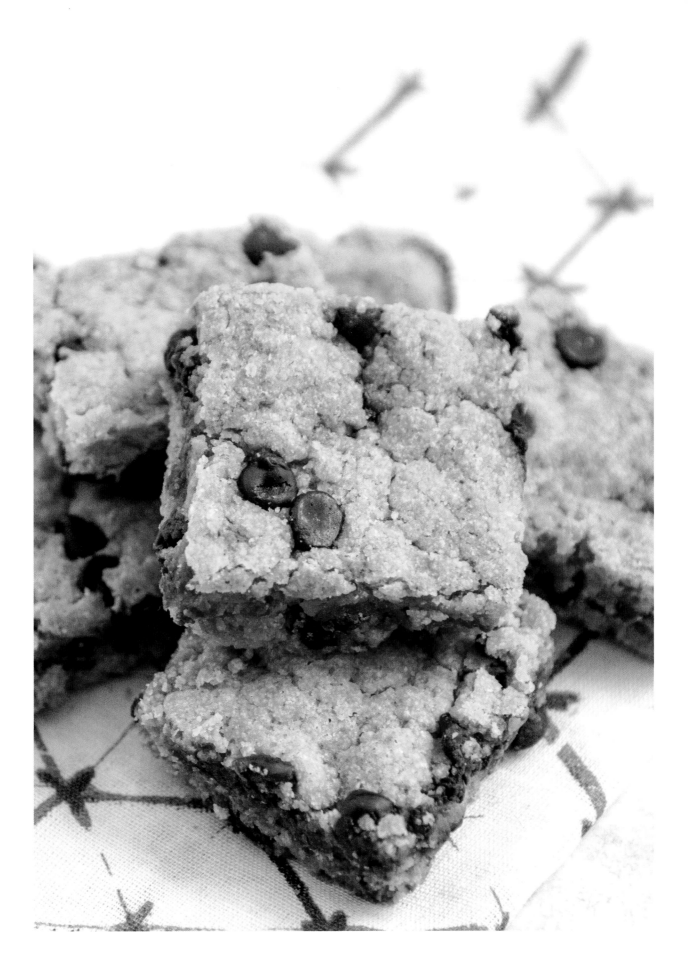

Fruit Pizza

yield: 8 servings

prep time: 15 minutes, plus 2 hours to chill

cook time: 14 minutes

Different variations of fruit pizza or, as some people call it, dessert pizza can be found at brunches and special events (especially showers!) in the South. The version I used to serve at gatherings I hosted had a sugar cookie crust. When I went keto, I really missed this dessert, and I wanted to make something similar that was low-carb. This version is just as delicious as the high-carb original, and it's so pretty! Feel free to use your favorite berries.

CRUST:

1¼ cups finely ground blanched almond flour

⅓ cup granular erythritol

1 teaspoon baking powder

1 large egg

5 tablespoons salted butter, softened

1 teaspoon vanilla extract

TOPPINGS:

5 ounces cream cheese (½ cup plus 2 tablespoons), softened

2 tablespoons granular erythritol

1 tablespoon heavy whipping cream

½ cup sliced fresh strawberries or whole raspberries

½ cup fresh blueberries

SPECIAL EQUIPMENT:
9-inch springform pan

1. Preheat the oven to 350°F and grease the bottom of a 9-inch springform pan.

2. Make the crust: In a small bowl, whisk together the almond flour, erythritol, and baking powder. In a medium-sized bowl, whisk the egg, then stir in the butter and vanilla extract. Stir in the flour mixture, a little at a time, until well combined.

3. Spread the crust mixture evenly in the prepared pan and bake for 12 to 14 minutes, until lightly browned on top and around the edges. Allow the crust to cool completely before releasing it from the pan.

4. While the crust is cooling, prepare the toppings: In a small bowl, use a spoon to beat the cream cheese, erythritol, and cream until completely combined. Spread evenly over the cooled crust. Garnish with fresh berries.

5. Cover and refrigerate the pizza for at least 2 hours before serving. Leftovers can be stored in an airtight container in the refrigerator for up to 2 days.

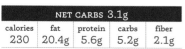

NET CARBS 3.1g				
calories	fat	protein	carbs	fiber
230	20.4g	5.6g	5.2g	2.1g

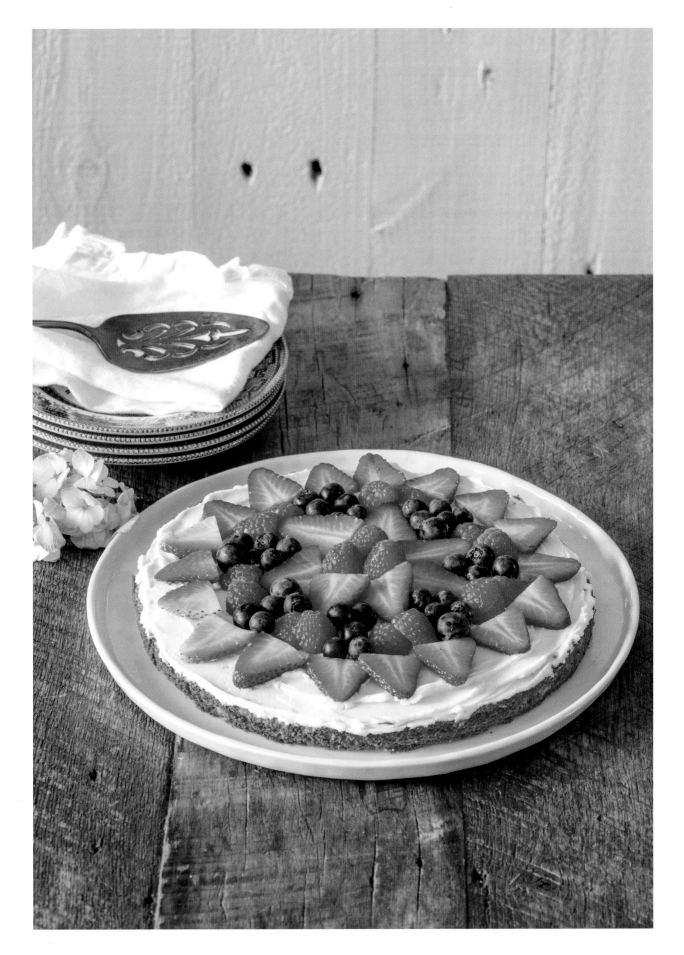

Peanut Butter Pie Bites with Chocolate Drizzle

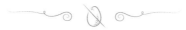

yield: 15 bites (3 per serving)

prep time: 10 minutes, plus 1 hour to freeze

Peanut butter pie is a popular dessert in the South. I always loved making mine with a chocolate crust. These pie bites are easier to make but still taste like peanut butter pie! I like to drizzle them with melted dark chocolate.

1 (8-ounce) package cream cheese, softened

½ cup natural peanut butter (smooth)

½ cup confectioners'-style erythritol

2 ounces dark chocolate (90% cacao), chopped

1. Line a sheet pan or tray with parchment paper.

2. In a medium-sized mixing bowl, cream together the cream cheese and peanut butter using a hand mixer on medium speed. When the mixture is creamy, slowly add the erythritol with the mixer running; continue mixing until all the ingredients are well combined and smooth.

3. In a small microwave-safe bowl, microwave the chocolate in 30-second increments, stirring after each increment, until the chocolate is melted and smooth.

4. Drop tablespoons of the peanut butter mixture onto the prepared pan. Use a fork to drizzle melted chocolate over each bite. Put the pan in the freezer for at least 1 hour before serving.

5. Take the bites out of the freezer and let them sit out for 10 minutes before eating. Leftovers can be stored in a resealable plastic bag or other airtight container in the freezer for up to a week.

NET CARBS 4.1g				
calories	fat	protein	carbs	fiber
309	27.1g	10g	7.8g	3.6g

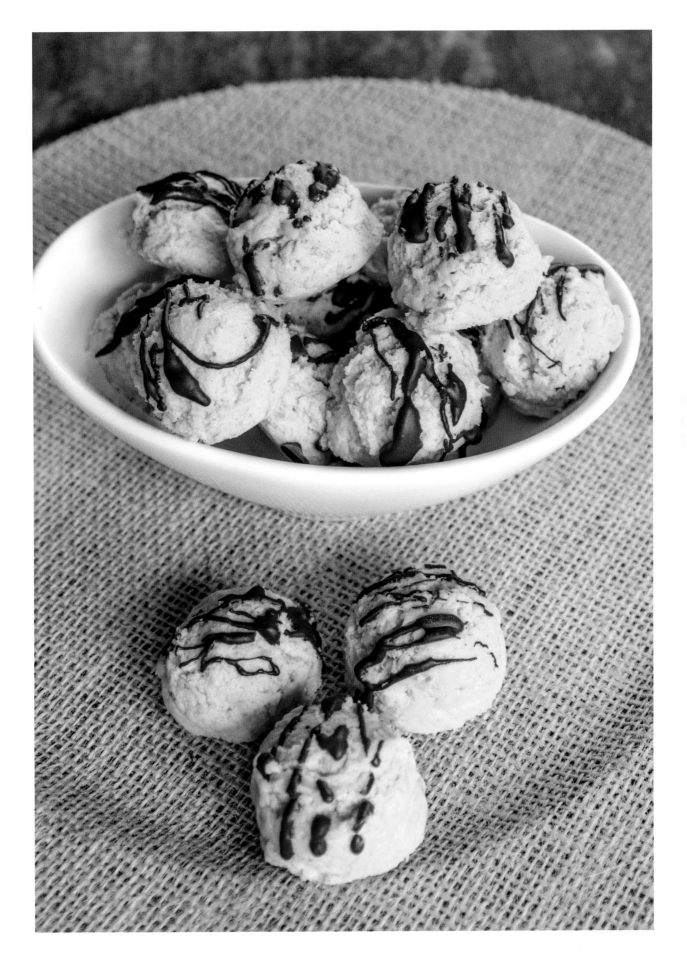

Chocolate Pecan Pie

yield: 8 servings
prep time: 10 minutes
cook time: 1 hour

I was so excited to create this keto version of the beloved pie I grew up eating. It's a Kentucky Derby party tradition. In some recipes, the filling is spiked with bourbon, but I opted to leave it out of this one. In my opinion, this pie is sort of a cross between a chocolate and a pecan pie—the best of both worlds!

2 large eggs

½ cup granular erythritol

¼ cup butter, melted but not hot

1 tablespoon coconut flour

½ teaspoon vanilla extract

¼ teaspoon salt

⅛ teaspoon liquid stevia

½ cup stevia-sweetened chocolate chips

½ cup chopped raw pecans

1 Almond Flour Crust (page 252), par-baked

1. Preheat the oven to 325°F.

2. In a medium-sized mixing bowl, whisk the eggs, erythritol, melted butter, coconut flour, vanilla, salt, and stevia until smooth. Fold in the chocolate chips and pecans and stir until well combined. Pour the batter into the par-baked crust.

3. Bake the pie for 50 to 60 minutes, until the filling is set and the top is golden brown. Let cool completely before serving. Leftovers can be covered and stored at room temperature for up to 3 days.

NET CARBS 3g				
calories	fat	protein	carbs	fiber
290	27.9g	8.4g	10.7g	5.4g

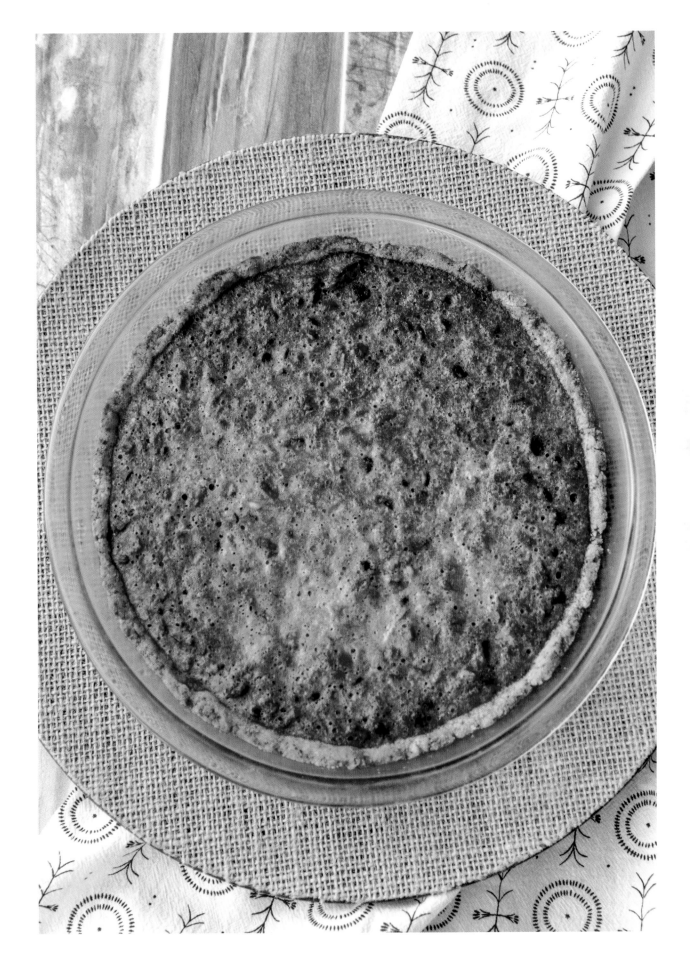

Praline Toasted Pecans

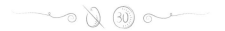

yield: 8 servings

prep time: 5 minutes

cook time: 20 minutes

My husband's parents in west Tennessee have pecan trees, so I always have pecans on hand. One of the things I used to make with them was sugared pecans. These pecans are even more delicious and don't contain any sugar! If you're a fan of sweet and salty, I suggest you sprinkle the finished pecans with a bit of sea salt.

2 cups raw pecan halves

½ cup packed brown sugar substitute (see Note)

2 tablespoons heavy whipping cream

¼ teaspoon vanilla extract

Medium-grind sea salt (optional)

1. Preheat the oven to 350°F. Line a sheet pan with parchment paper.

2. Place all the ingredients in a medium-sized mixing bowl and stir with a spoon until the pecans are evenly coated.

3. Spread the pecans evenly on the prepared pan and bake for 10 minutes, then stir and bake for 10 more minutes, or until golden brown. Sprinkle with sea salt, if desired. Allow to cool completely before serving. Leftover pecans can be stored in an airtight container at room temperature for up to 2 weeks.

Note:

You can use unflavored granular sweetener if you wish, but the brown sugar flavor is especially tasty in this recipe.

NET CARBS 1.3g				
calories	fat	protein	carbs	fiber
202	21g	2.6g	3.9g	2.6g

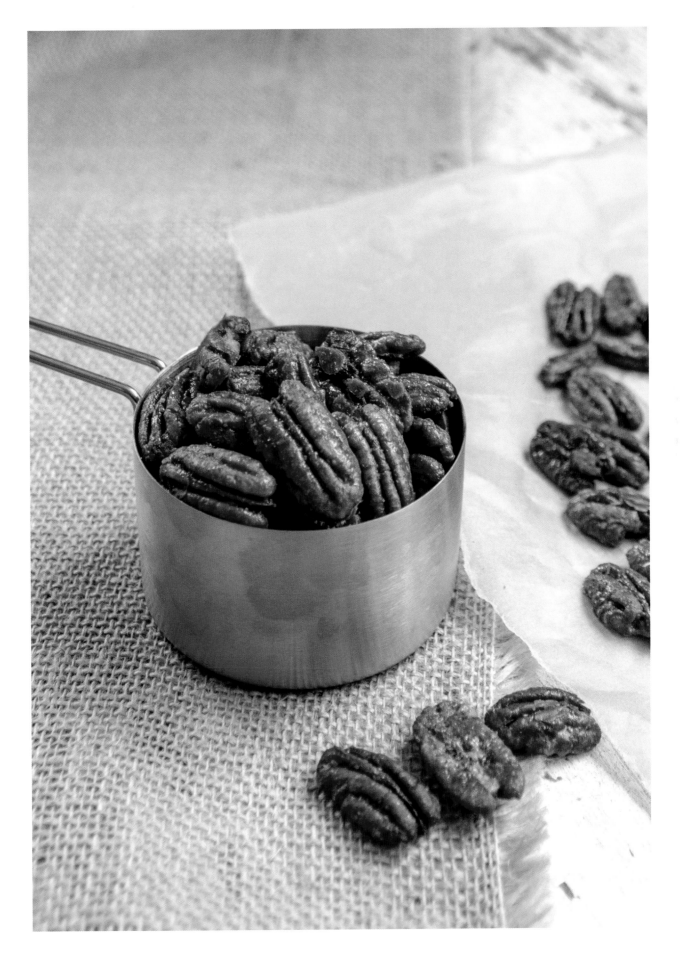

One-Bowl Butter Cookies

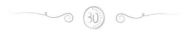

yield: 12 cookies (2 per serving)

prep time: 5 minutes

cook time: 14 minutes

½ cup (1 stick) salted butter, softened

1½ cups finely ground blanched almond flour

¼ teaspoon salt

½ cup granular erythritol

½ teaspoon vanilla extract

1 large egg

⅛ teaspoon liquid stevia

These cookies are the easiest I've ever made, and they sacrifice nothing in flavor. We love them just like this, but you could experiment by adding different flavor extracts.

1. Preheat the oven to 350°F. Line a baking sheet with parchment paper.

2. Put all the ingredients in a medium-sized mixing bowl. Using a hand mixer, slowly blend on low speed, then increase the speed to medium and continue mixing until everything is well combined.

3. Using a small cookie scoop, scoop the dough onto the prepared pan, leaving 2 inches of space between the cookies. Use the back of a fork to press crisscrosses on each cookie.

4. Bake for 12 to 14 minutes, until the cookies start to turn light brown around the edges. Allow to cool completely before removing from the pan. The cookies will continue to firm up as they cool. Leftovers can be stored in an airtight container at room temperature for up to a week.

Note:
You also can use a stand mixer fitted with a dough hook attachment to mix the cookie dough.

NET CARBS 1.7g				
calories	fat	protein	carbs	fiber
297	28.6g	2.5g	4.2g	2.5g

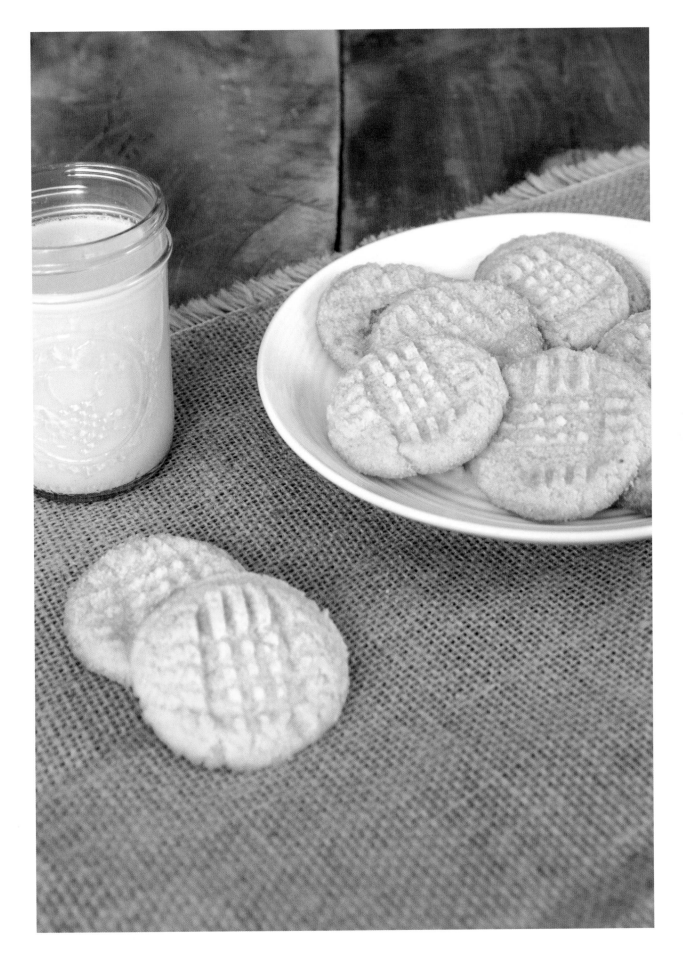

Strawberry Shortcakes

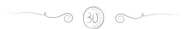

yield: 6 servings

prep time: 10 minutes

cook time: 15 minutes

In the South, we serve anything with (or on!) biscuits—yes, even dessert! Whether you call these shortcake-style biscuits or biscuit-y shortcakes, you will love them. Though fresh strawberries and whipped cream are the classic topping combination for these sweet little biscuitlike cakes, you may find more uses for them—or even eat them plain!

1½ cups fresh strawberries

¾ cup finely ground blanched almond flour

1 teaspoon baking powder

⅛ teaspoon salt

1 large egg

⅓ cup granular erythritol

2 tablespoons heavy whipping cream

2 tablespoons salted butter, melted but not hot

½ teaspoon vanilla extract

1½ cups Whipped Cream (page 254), for serving

1. Preheat the oven to 375°F. Line a baking sheet with parchment paper.

2. Hull and slice the strawberries and set aside.

3. In a small bowl, whisk together the almond flour, baking powder, and salt.

4. In a medium-sized mixing bowl, whisk the egg, then stir in the erythritol, cream, melted butter, and vanilla extract. While stirring, slowly add the dry ingredients; continue stirring until well blended.

5. Drop spoonfuls of the batter onto the prepared baking sheet, spacing the shortcakes 2 inches apart, to make a total of 6 shortcakes. Bake for 13 to 15 minutes, until the shortcakes are golden brown on the tops and a toothpick or tester inserted in the middle of a shortcake comes out clean. Allow to completely cool on the pan.

6. To serve, top the shortcakes with whipped cream and the sliced strawberries. Leftover shortcakes can be stored in an airtight container in the refrigerator for up to 5 days.

NET CARBS 3.3g				
calories	fat	protein	carbs	fiber
154	13.1g	4g	5.3g	2g

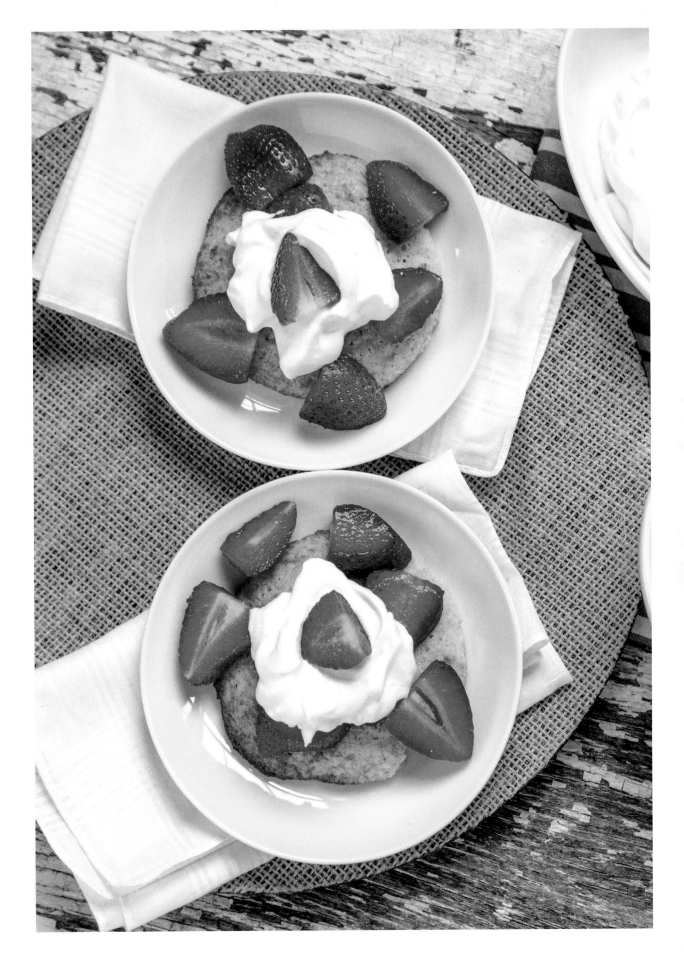

Quick Blackberry Cobbler for Two

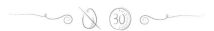

yield: 2 servings
prep time: 5 minutes
cook time: 2 minutes

I have a special place in my heart for blackberry cobbler. In Kentucky, when blackberries were in season, my mom and I would walk up the road from our house and pick a bunch of them. We would come directly home, and she would make a cobbler. I've shared this quick little recipe with her, and she approves. She has even made it with strawberries!

1½ cups fresh blackberries

¼ teaspoon liquid stevia (see Note)

¼ teaspoon vanilla extract

¼ cup finely ground blanched almond flour

¼ cup (½ stick) cold salted butter, cubed

½ teaspoon baking powder

Whipped Cream (page 254), for serving (optional)

1. Grease a 2-cup microwave-safe baking dish.

2. In a small bowl, gently combine the blackberries, stevia, and vanilla extract, then pour the mixture into the prepared baking dish.

3. In a small bowl, use a fork to stir together the almond flour and baking powder, then add the butter and continue stirring with the fork until a crumbly mixture forms. Sprinkle the mixture evenly over the blackberries.

4. Microwave for 1½ to 2 minutes, checking every 30 seconds, until the blackberries are bubbly and the topping is lightly browned; microwave cook times vary according to wattage. Allow the cobbler to cool for 10 minutes. Serve with whipped cream, if desired.

Note:

If your blackberries are particularly tart, you might want to increase the amount of sweetener.

NET CARBS 5.8g				
calories	fat	protein	carbs	fiber
328	30g	4.3g	12.8g	7g

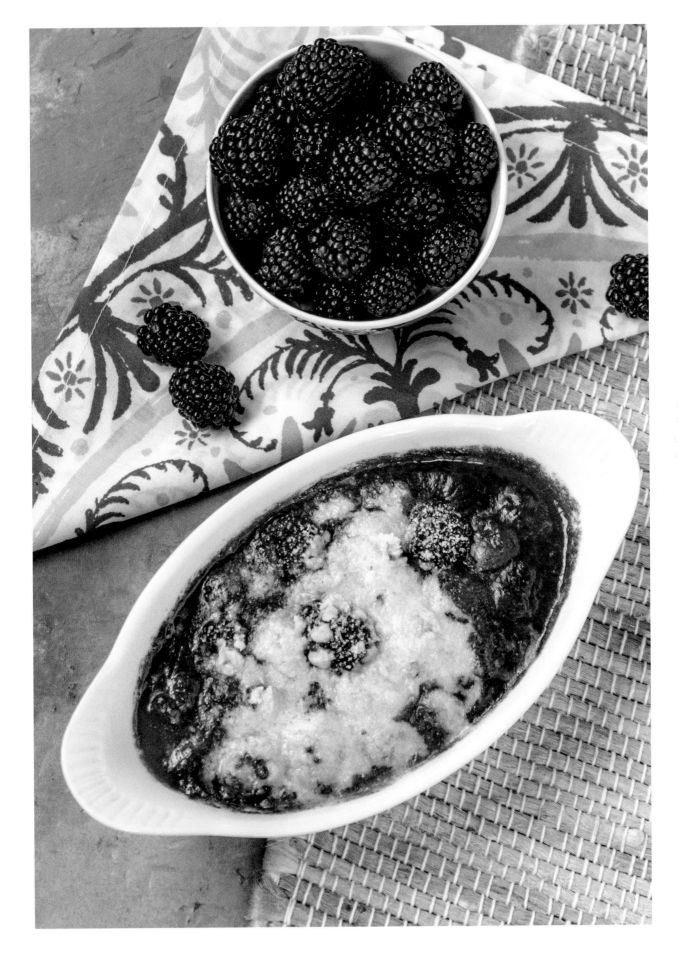

Easy Truffles

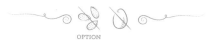

yield: 18 truffles (1 per serving)

prep time: 15 minutes, plus 2 hours to chill

Who knew truffles could be so easy to make? And they're pretty, too! Experiment with different toppings. If you tire of cocoa powder or shredded coconut, try a coating of crushed nuts. I personally gravitate toward pecans, but that is simply because pecans are the nut of choice here in the South when it comes to desserts (and because I love their buttery rich flavor). You can also add flavor extracts to these truffles.

1 cup sugar-free chocolate chips

½ cup heavy whipping cream

SUGGESTED COATINGS:

Cocoa powder

Unsweetened shredded coconut

Crushed nuts (raw or roasted) of choice

1. Put the chocolate chips in small bowl.

2. In a small saucepan over low heat, bring the cream to a simmer.

3. Pour the hot cream over the chocolate. Allow to sit for a few minutes, until the chocolate begins to melt, then stir until smooth. Allow to cool, then refrigerate the mixture for 2 hours.

4. Line a small sheet pan or tray with parchment paper.

5. To make the truffles, scoop a teaspoon-sized ball of the chocolate mixture. Quickly roll it between the palms of your hands. Then roll it in the coating of your choice and place the ball on the lined pan. Repeat with the rest of the truffle mixture and coating.

6. Refrigerate for at least 1 hour before serving. Allow the truffles to sit out for 10 minutes to soften before eating. Store in an airtight container in the refrigerator for up to a week.

NET CARBS 1.49g				
calories	fat	protein	carbs	fiber
149	5.5g	0.8g	6.1g	2.6g

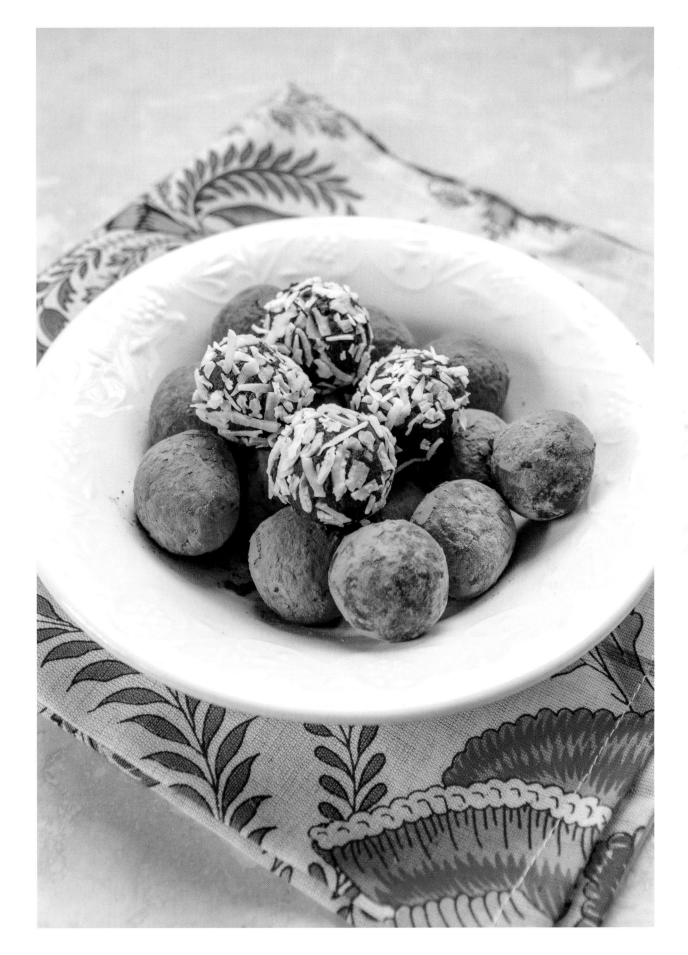

Kentucky Bourbon Balls

yield: 12 balls (1 per serving)

prep time: 20 minutes, plus
1 hour to chill

cook time: 3 minutes

Bourbon balls are a true Southern delicacy. Owing to Kentucky's many bourbon distilleries, they may be particularly popular there, in my home state. Bourbon balls often found their way onto our holiday tables when I was growing up. My husband, from Tennessee, grew up eating them, too. Every holiday season, his grandma would make several batches. As she made each batch, she would take a nip or two of bourbon, and the last batches always ended up being a bit "stiffer" than the first ones!

½ cup (1 stick) salted butter, softened

1 cup confectioners'-style erythritol

3 tablespoons bourbon (see Note)

½ teaspoon vanilla extract

¼ cup chopped raw pecans

¾ cup sugar-free chocolate chips

1 tablespoon avocado oil

12 raw pecan halves, for garnish

SPECIAL EQUIPMENT
(optional):
12 individual foil candy cups

1. Using a hand mixer on medium speed, beat the butter and erythritol until pale yellow and fluffy. Add the bourbon, vanilla extract, and pecans and stir until well combined. Place in the refrigerator for 30 minutes, until chilled and easier to shape.

2. Place the chocolate chips and oil in a small microwave-safe bowl. Microwave in 30-second increments, stirring after each increment, until melted and smooth.

3. Have on hand 12 foil candy cups or line a tray with parchment paper. Take the pecan mixture out of the refrigerator and roll 1-tablespoon scoops into 1-inch balls. Using a spoon, dip each ball into the melted chocolate to coat, then place in the candy cups or on the lined tray. Top each ball with a pecan half.

4. Place back in the refrigerator for at least 1 hour before serving. Allow the balls to sit out for 10 minutes to soften before eating. Store in an airtight container in the refrigerator for up to 2 weeks.

Note:
For best results, use a high-quality bourbon with a smooth flavor. In general, you should use a bourbon that you enjoy sipping. Because these confections are not cooked, they are very slightly boozy and should only be served to adults.

NET CARBS 1.08g				
calories	fat	protein	carbs	fiber
117	11.5g	0.8g	4.8g	2.2g

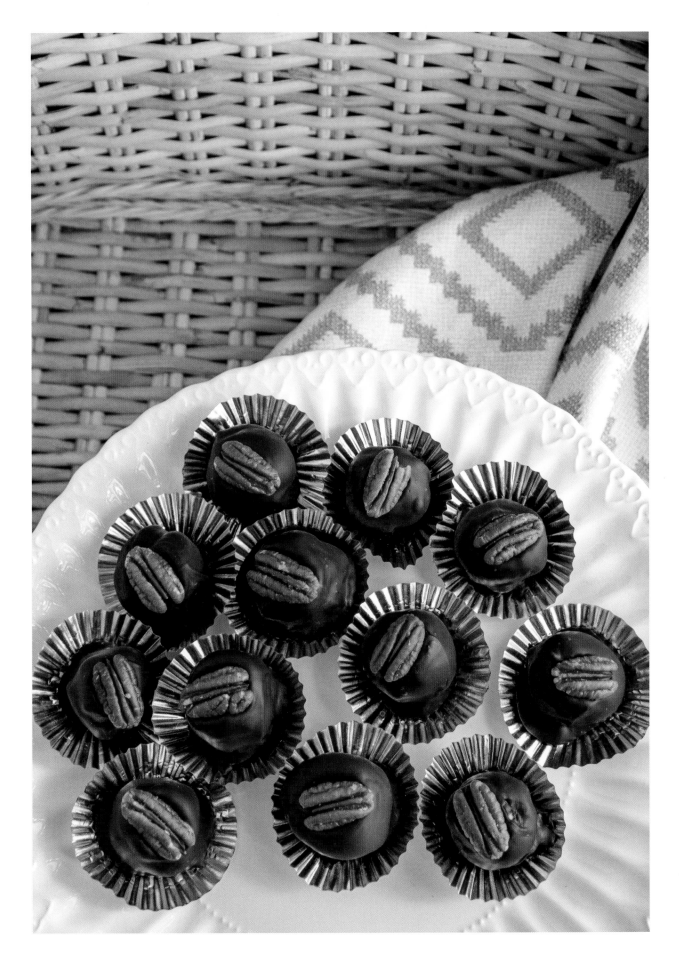

Chocolate Pudding

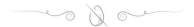

yield: 2 servings

prep time: 10 minutes, plus 2 hours to chill

A yummy and easy pudding for two! Unlike a traditional pudding that's thickened by slowly cooking egg yolks until they develop a custardy texture, this pudding is thickened with chia seeds, and very little hands-on prep time is required. Along with being a good thickener, chia seeds are an excellent source of protein, fiber, and healthy fats.

1 cup unsweetened almond milk

¼ cup cocoa powder

2 tablespoons chia seeds

2 tablespoons heavy whipping cream

2 tablespoons granular erythritol

FOR GARNISH (optional):

Whipped Cream (page 254)

Shaved ultra-dark chocolate (about 90% cacao)

1. Place all the ingredients in a blender. Blend on high speed until the mixture starts to thicken; this will take at least 2 minutes.

2. Pour the pudding into a 2-cup dish. Refrigerate for at least 2 hours before serving. Garnish the pudding with whipped cream and dark chocolate shavings, if desired.

Note:

For a nut-free pudding, you can use unsweetened coconut milk in place of almond milk.

NET CARBS 3.5g				
calories	fat	protein	carbs	fiber
137	11.2g	4.6g	10.7g	7.1g

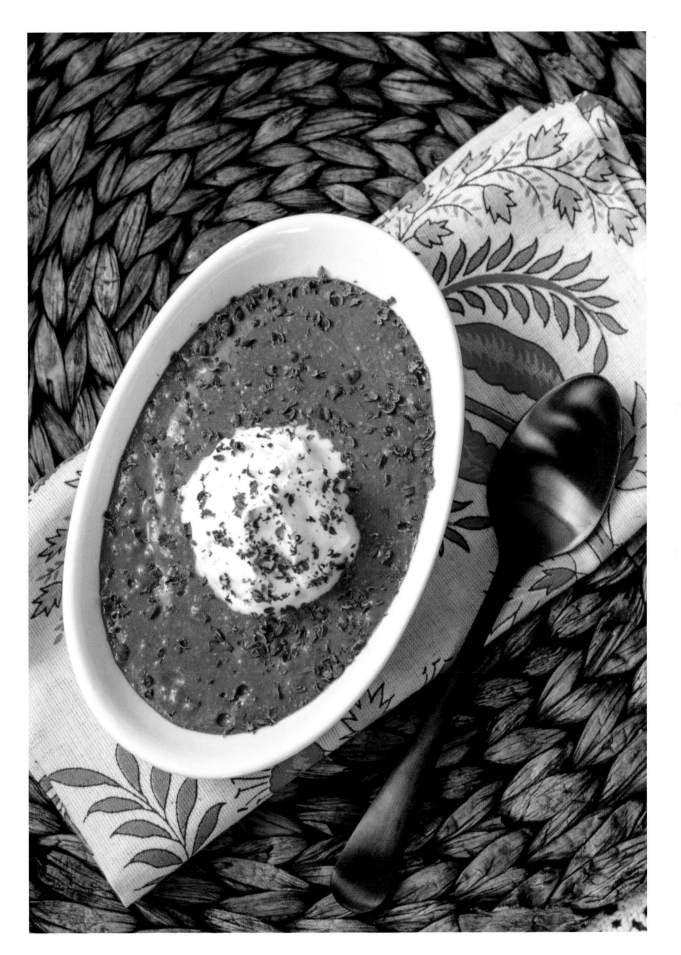

Dark Chocolate Coconut Fat Bombs

yield: 8 fat bombs
(2 per serving)

prep time: 10 minutes, plus
2 hours to freeze

1 cup sugar-free chocolate chips

¼ cup (½ stick) salted butter

1 cup unsweetened coconut flakes, plus extra for garnish if desired

SPECIAL EQUIPMENT:
8 individual foil candy cups, or a silicone candy mold with 1-inch cavities

These coconut-filled fat bombs couldn't be any easier to make! My daughter said they remind her of a Mounds candy bar. They really do! If you're fonder of the Almond Joy version, you could add almonds to the tops of these.

1. In a small microwave-safe bowl, microwave the chocolate chips in 20-second increments, stirring after each increment, until the chocolate has melted. Add the butter and stir until the butter has melted. Stir in the coconut until thoroughly combined.

2. Pour the mixture into 8 foil candy cups or 8 cavities of a silicone candy mold, filling them almost to the top. Garnish with extra coconut, if desired.

3. Freeze for at least 2 hours. Store in an airtight container in the refrigerator for up to a week.

	NET CARBS 1.4g			
calories	fat	protein	carbs	fiber
165	13.9g	3.9g	4.4g	3.1g

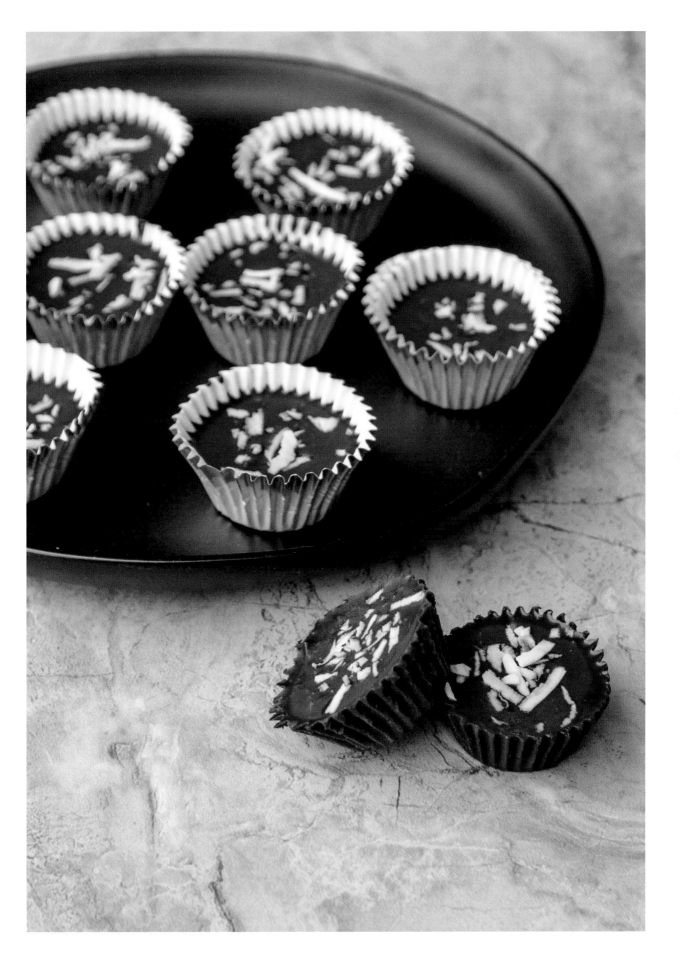

Glazed Coconut Bundt Cake

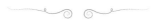

yield: 10 servings
prep time: 30 minutes
cook time: 55 minutes

I love my Bundt pans, and they had been underused since I started the keto life, so I was excited to create this decadent dessert. Not only does the cake itself make use of coconut oil and coconut flour, but it's also topped with toasted coconut flakes, a beloved Southern dessert ingredient. Don't skip the step of toasting the coconut; it really adds a special touch.

CAKE:

2 cups finely ground blanched almond flour

¼ cup coconut flour

¾ cup granular erythritol

2 teaspoons baking powder

½ teaspoon salt

5 large eggs

½ cup (1 stick) salted butter, softened

¼ cup coconut oil, softened

2 teaspoons vanilla extract

1 cup unsweetened coconut flakes

GARNISH:

½ cup unsweetened coconut flakes

GLAZE:

½ cup confectioners'-style erythritol

¼ cup heavy whipping cream

¼ teaspoon vanilla extract

1. Preheat the oven to 350°F. Grease a 12-cup Bundt pan with butter.

2. In a medium-sized bowl, whisk the almond flour, coconut flour, granular erythritol, baking powder, and salt. In a large mixing bowl, use a hand mixer on low speed to blend the eggs, butter, coconut oil, and vanilla extract. With the mixer on low speed, slowly blend in the flour mixture. Use a spoon to stir in the coconut flakes.

3. Spoon the batter into the prepared pan, then smooth the top. Bake for 45 minutes, until a toothpick or tester inserted into the middle comes out clean. Place the pan on a wire rack to cool completely. Lower the oven temperature to 325°F for toasting the coconut.

4. Make the toasted coconut garnish: Line a sheet pan with parchment paper. Spread the coconut in a thin layer on the prepared pan. Bake for 5 minutes, stir the coconut, then return to the oven and bake until golden brown. It shouldn't take more than another 5 minutes; keep a close eye on it, as coconut can burn quickly. Remove the coconut from the pan and allow to cool.

5. Make the glaze: Put the confectioners'-style erythritol, cream, and vanilla extract in a small bowl and stir until smooth.

6. To serve, gently loosen the sides of the cooled cake from the pan with a knife and turn it onto a cake plate. Pour the glaze evenly over the cake. Garnish the cake with the toasted coconut. The cake can be kept covered on the counter for a day. Leftovers can be stored in an airtight container in the refrigerator for up to a week.

NET CARBS 3.1g				
calories	fat	protein	carbs	fiber
361	31.4g	10.2g	7.5g	4.4g

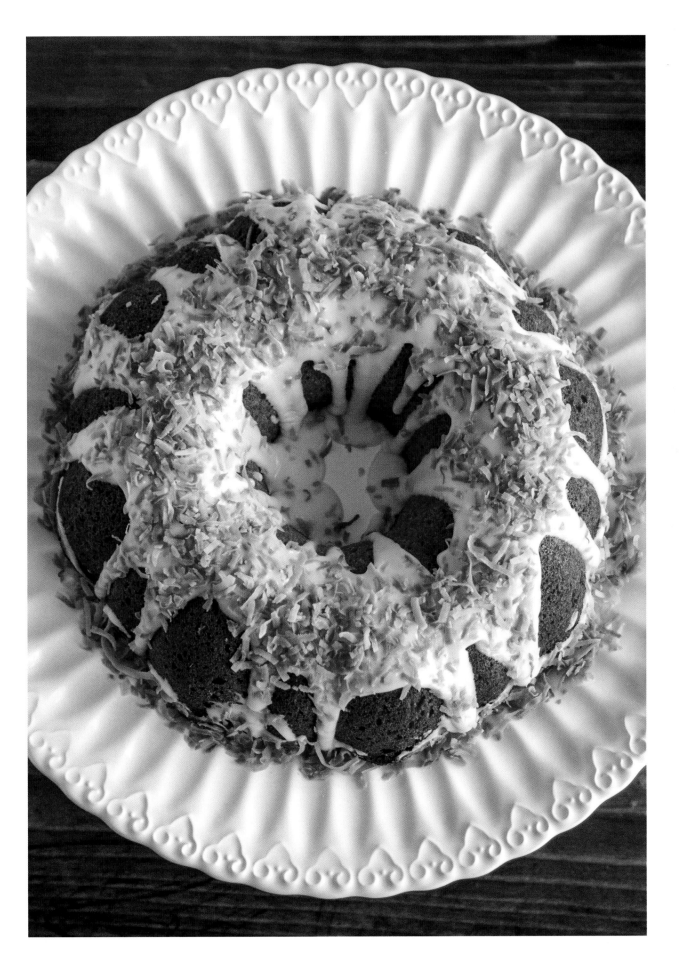

Pumpkin Pie

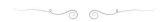

yield: 8 servings
prep time: 15 minutes
cook time: 50 minutes

Pumpkin-everything season is my favorite. It's the time of year when pumpkin-flavored items start showing up everywhere. Truthfully, I like pumpkin flavor enough to have it at any time of the year. This year, you don't have to miss out on having pumpkin pie on the Thanksgiving table.

2 large eggs

1 (15-ounce) can pumpkin puree

½ cup granular erythritol

1 tablespoon pumpkin pie spice

1 teaspoon ground cinnamon

½ teaspoon salt

¾ cup heavy whipping cream

1 Almond Flour Crust (page 252), par-baked

1. Preheat the oven to 350°F.

2. In a medium-sized mixing bowl, whisk the eggs. Stir in the pumpkin puree, erythritol, pumpkin pie spice, cinnamon, and salt with a spoon until well blended. While stirring, slowly pour in the cream; continue stirring until it's completely combined with the pumpkin mixture.

3. Pour the filling into the par-baked crust. Cover the edge of the crust with a narrow piece of aluminum foil to keep it from burning; remove the foil midway through baking. Bake until the filling is set, doesn't jiggle, and is lightly browned on top, 45 to 50 minutes. Allow to cool completely before cutting and serving. Leftover pie can be covered and stored in the refrigerator for up to 5 days.

Note:

This pie can also be baked without a crust so that it's a crustless pumpkin pie. Simply pour the filling into a greased 9-inch pie pan and bake as described above.

NET CARBS 2.2g				
calories	fat	protein	carbs	fiber
250	23.6g	5.4g	4.1g	1.9g

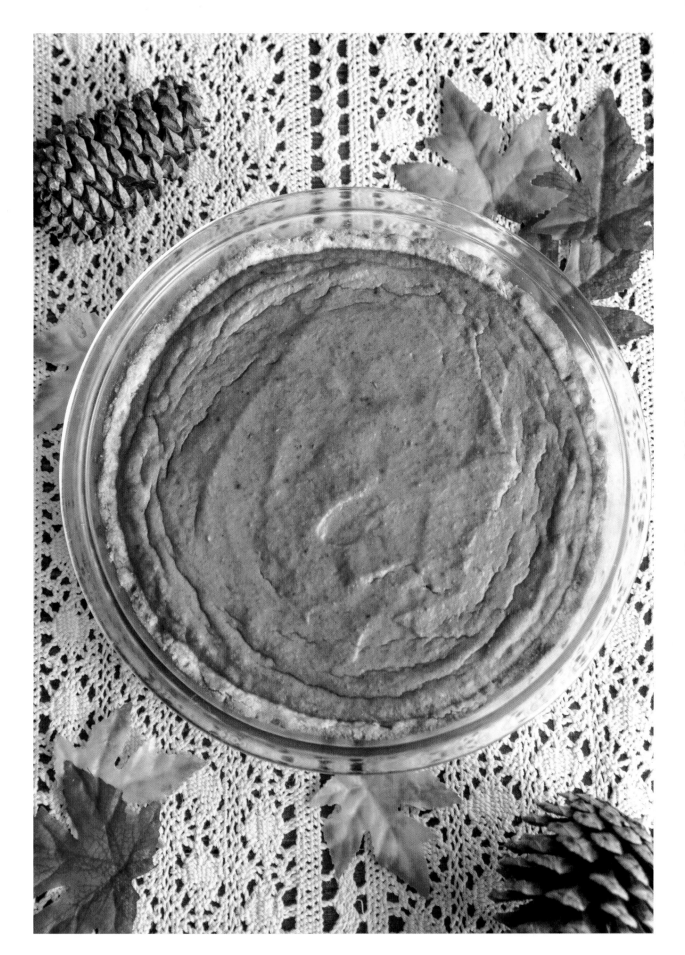

Almond Flour Crust

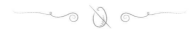

yield: one 9-inch pie crust (8 servings)

prep time: 10 minutes, plus 30 minutes to chill

cook time: 12 to 15 minutes

1¼ cups finely ground blanched almond flour

1 teaspoon granular erythritol (omit for savory crust)

¼ teaspoon salt

¼ cup (½ stick) cold salted butter, cubed

1 to 2 tablespoons cold water

I love making crustless pies, but sometimes you crave a good crust. This easy-to-make crust is multipurpose: you can use it for desserts or for savory pies. It is more fragile than a crust made with regular flour, so use it right away.

1. In a medium-sized mixing bowl, whisk together the flour, erythritol (if using), and salt. Add the butter and use a pastry blender or fork to break up the butter until the mixture resembles coarse crumbs. Add the water 1 tablespoon at a time until the dough is moistened and you can form it into a ball. Wrap the ball of dough in plastic wrap and refrigerate for 30 minutes.

2. Preheat the oven to 350°F. Grease a 9-inch pie plate with oil or butter.

3. Using your hands, press the dough evenly across the bottom and up the sides of the prepared pie plate. If it gets sticky, dampen your fingers with water. Use a fork to lightly prick the bottom of the crust several times.

4. Par-bake the crust for 12 to 15 minutes, until light golden brown. Let cool before filling and baking.

NET CARBS 1.1g				
calories	fat	protein	carbs	fiber
147	13.8g	3.3g	2.7g	1.6g

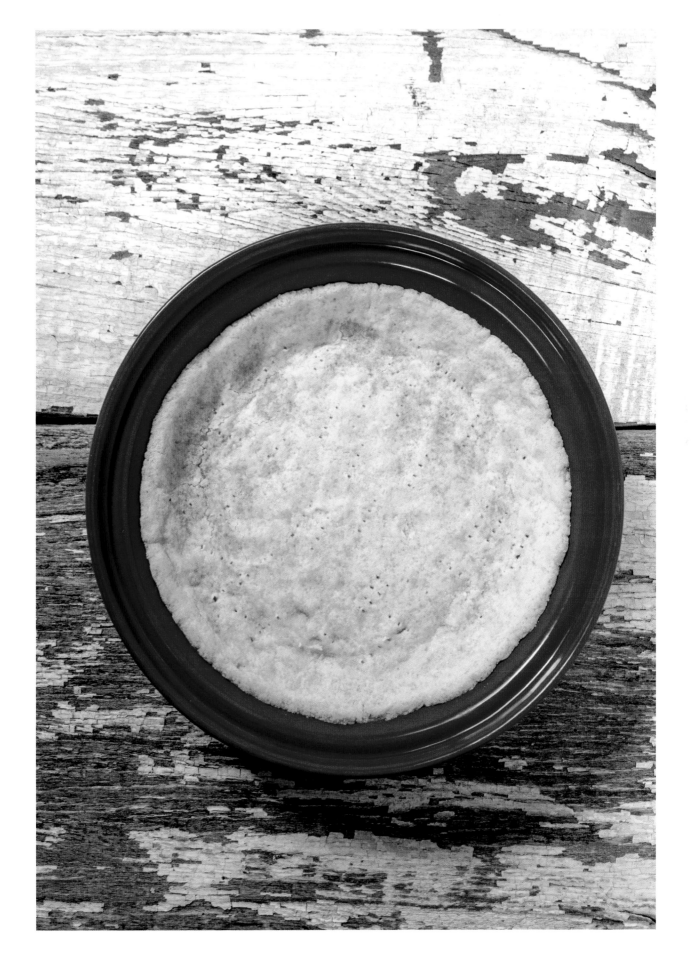

Whipped Cream

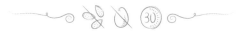

yield: 2 cups (¼ cup per serving)

prep time: 5 minutes

1 cup heavy whipping cream

2 tablespoons granular erythritol

1 teaspoon vanilla extract

There's nothing quite like homemade whipped cream, and it's a breeze to make. It goes with all your favorite desserts, and it's even good all by itself!

Place the ingredients in a large mixing bowl. Use a hand mixer or stand mixer to blend until stiff peaks form. Whipped cream is best if used the same day it's made, but leftovers can be stored in an airtight container in the refrigerator for up to 3 days.

NET CARBS 1.6g				
calories	fat	protein	carbs	fiber
220	22.8g	1.1g	1.6g	0g

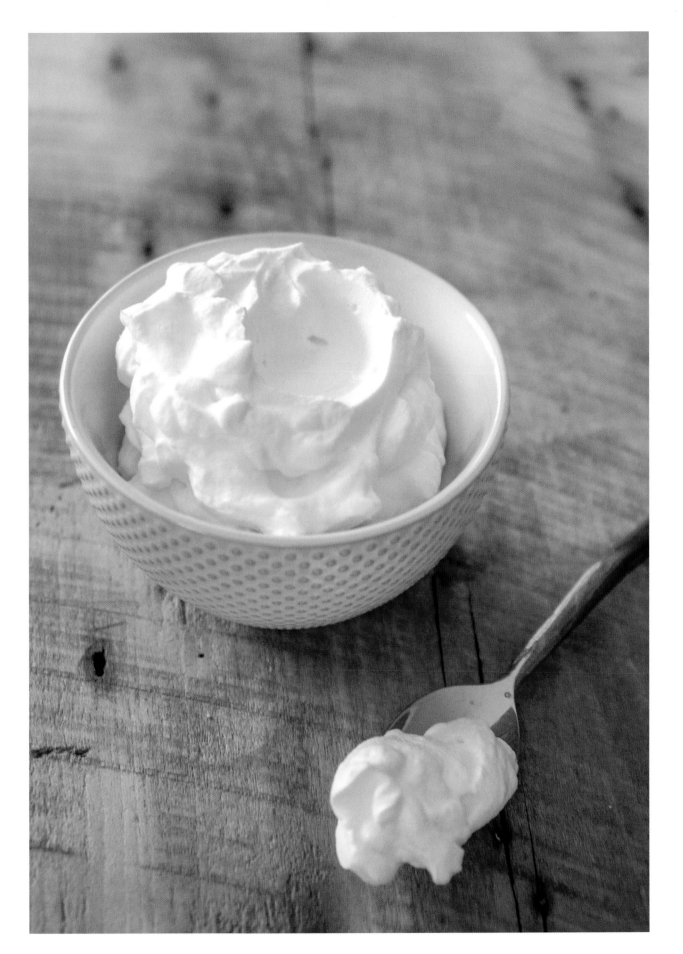

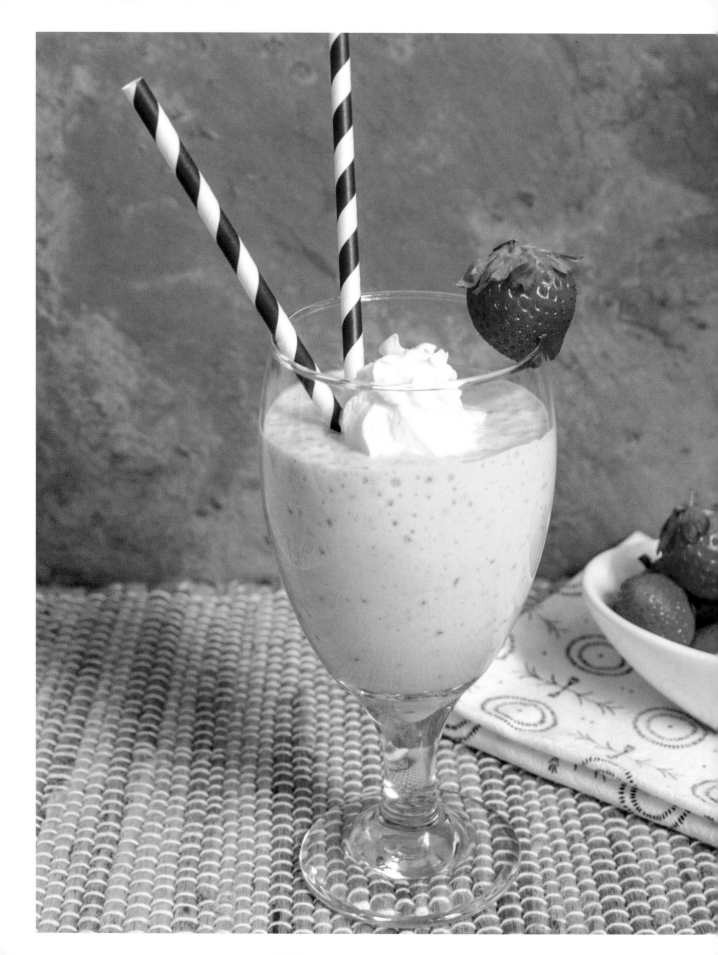

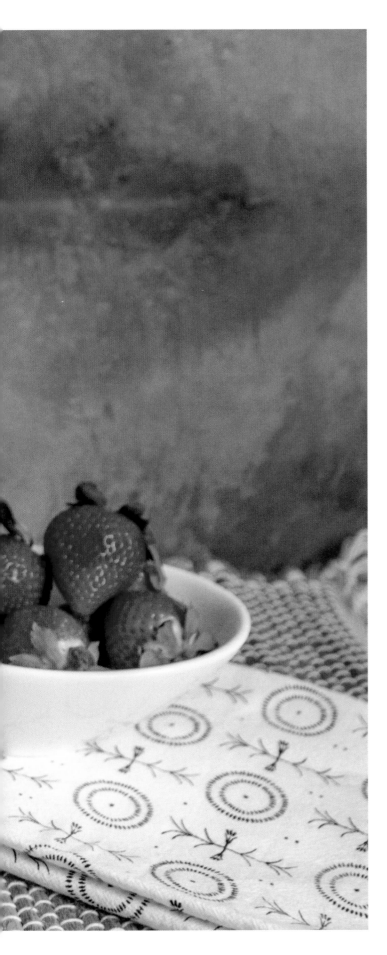

Drinks

Strawberry Milkshake

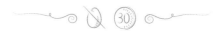

yield: 1 serving

prep time: 5 minutes

4 medium-sized cold or frozen strawberries, plus 1 fresh berry for garnish if desired

¾ cup unsweetened almond milk

¼ cup heavy whipping cream

1½ teaspoons granular erythritol

¼ teaspoon vanilla extract

¼ teaspoon xanthan gum (see Note)

Whipped Cream (page 254), for garnish (optional)

Who doesn't love a milkshake? My first job was at Dairy Queen, so I know a thing or two about making milkshakes! You won't believe how close this version tastes to a real strawberry milkshake; the cream makes it taste so good.

Put all the ingredients in a blender and blend on high speed until smooth and creamy, about 1 minute. Pour into a 16-ounce glass and serve immediately. Garnish with whipped cream and a strawberry, if desired.

Note:

If you don't have xanthan gum, you can leave it out, but it thickens the milkshake and gives it the perfect texture.

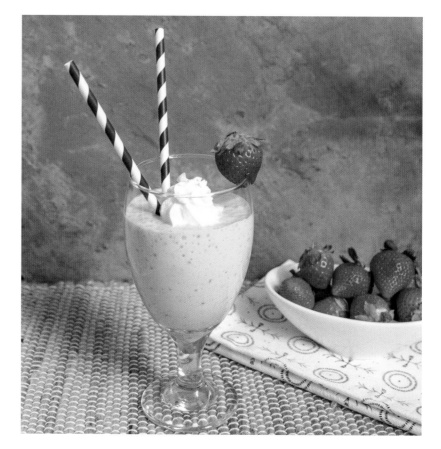

NET CARBS 4.8g				
calories	fat	protein	carbs	fiber
254	24.4g	2.1g	6.6g	1.8g

Keto Berry Smoothie

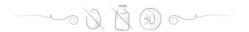

yield: 1 serving

prep time: 5 minutes

A lot of people think you can't have smoothies on keto, but it's actually really easy to make a great low-carb, high-fat smoothie.

1 cup baby spinach leaves

1 cup unsweetened almond milk

½ cup ice

½ cup fresh blackberries or other berries of choice, plus extra for garnish if desired

¼ cup raw pecan halves

1 tablespoon MCT oil

¼ teaspoon vanilla extract

⅛ teaspoon liquid stevia

Unsweetened coconut flakes, for garnish

Place all the ingredients in a blender and blend on high speed until smooth and creamy, about 1 minute. Pour into a 16-ounce glass and serve immediately. Garnish with coconut flakes and berries, if desired.

Note:

You can experiment with a variety of nuts, berries, and extracts to create different smoothie flavors.

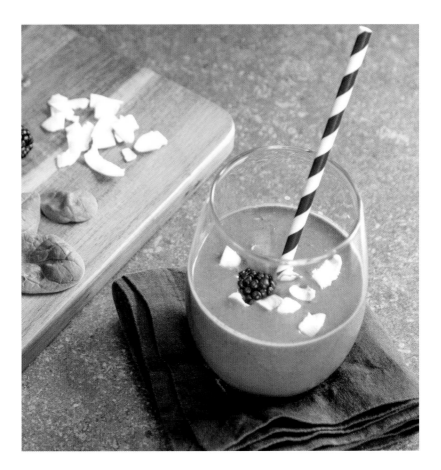

NET CARBS 5.5g				
calories	fat	protein	carbs	fiber
360	34.8g	5.3g	13.1g	7.6g

Keto Sweet Tea

yield: 8 servings

prep time: 5 minutes, plus 20 minutes to steep

cook time: 10 minutes

1 gallon filtered water, divided

4 family-sized bags black tea

¾ cup granular erythritol

5 drops liquid stevia

Ice, for serving

Lemon wedges, for garnish (optional)

Southern as sweet tea! Growing up in the South, I thought everyone liked their tea sweet. If you prefer yours a little less sweet, decrease the amount of erythritol to ½ cup.

1. In a large saucepan, bring 2 quarts of water to a boil. Remove from the heat and add the tea bags. Allow to steep for 20 minutes. Pour the other 2 quarts of water into a gallon-sized pitcher.

2. Remove the tea bags and squeeze them. Stir in both sweeteners until completely dissolved. Pour the concentrated tea mixture into the pitcher and stir to combine.

3. Serve over ice in tall 16-ounce glasses garnished with lemon wedges. Store in the refrigerator for up to a week.

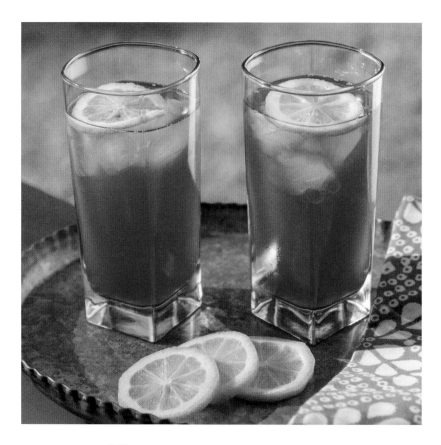

NET CARBS 0g				
calories	fat	protein	carbs	fiber
0	0g	0g	0g	0g

Hot Chocolate

yield: 1 serving
prep time: 5 minutes
cook time: 10 minutes

Sometimes I like to have a cup of hot chocolate at night. I used to drink lots of the boxed kind. This low-carb version is easy to make and keeps me on plan!

1 cup unsweetened almond milk

¼ cup heavy whipping cream

1 tablespoon cocoa powder

1 tablespoon granular erythritol

⅛ teaspoon vanilla extract

FOR SERVING (optional):

Whipped Cream (page 254)

Sugar-free chocolate chips

Heat the almond milk, cream, cocoa powder, and erythritol in a small saucepan over low heat. Stir until the cocoa and sweetener are dissolved and all the ingredients are well blended and hot. Remove from the heat and stir in the vanilla extract. Pour the hot chocolate into a 12-ounce mug and top with whipped cream and chocolate chips, if desired.

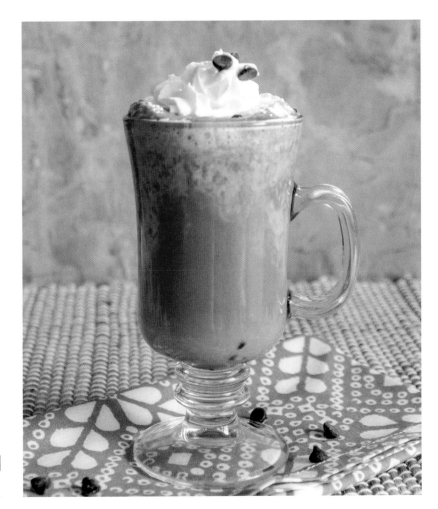

NET CARBS 4g				
calories	fat	protein	carbs	fiber
283	27.2g	3.8g	6.2g	2.2g

Lemonade for One

yield: 1 serving
prep time: 5 minutes

Nothing tastes quite like a glass of fresh lemonade on a hot day. I love this single-serving lemonade because it's easy to make a quick glass for yourself. However, you easily can double or quadruple the recipe to share with a friend (or two).

¼ cup hot water

1 tablespoon granular erythritol

Juice of 1 lemon

¾ cup cold water

Lemon slice, for garnish

In a 16-ounce glass, stir together the hot water and erythritol until the erythritol is dissolved. Stir in the lemon juice and cold water. Fill the glass with ice and garnish with a lemon slice.

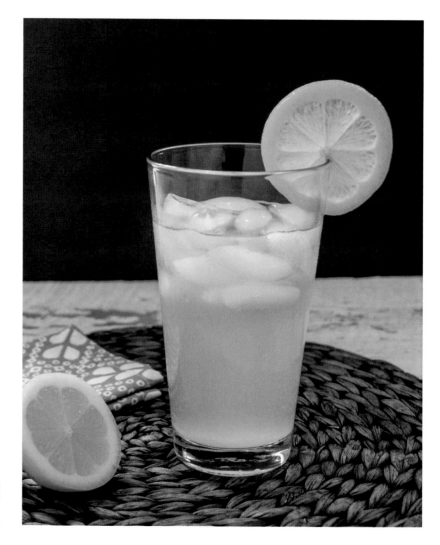

NET CARBS 3.2g				
calories	fat	protein	carbs	fiber
11	0.1g	0.2g	3.3g	0.1g

Bulletproof Coffee

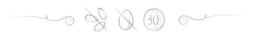

yield: 1 serving

prep time: 5 minutes

1 cup hot coffee

1 tablespoon MCT oil

1 tablespoon salted butter

1 scoop unflavored collagen peptides

Liquid stevia

Here's a basic recipe for the ever-popular fatty keto coffee! Feel free to add your favorite flavors to dress it up. A dash of cinnamon is always a good choice.

Put all the ingredients, except the stevia, in a blender. Blend until frothy, 30 to 60 seconds. Sweeten with stevia to taste. Pour into a 12-ounce mug and serve immediately.

Note:

You can add different sugar-free flavorings and extracts to your coffee. Cocoa powder is a good option to make a mocha-flavored version.

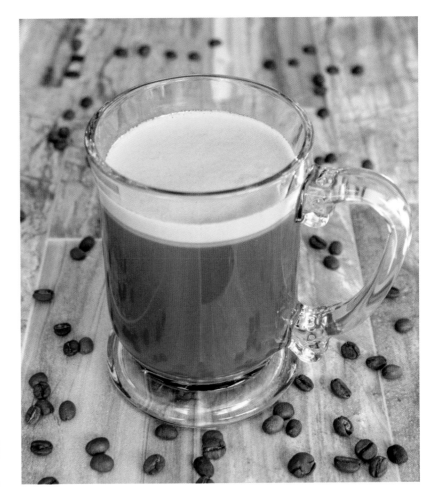

NET CARBS 0g				
calories	fat	protein	carbs	fiber
245	25.2g	6.4g	0g	0g

Southern Boiled Custard

yield: 4 servings
prep time: 10 minutes
cook time: 30 minutes

When I was growing up, it was tradition to have boiled custard at Christmastime. My mamaw and her sister would make gallons of it, as it was very popular in our family. This isn't a custard that you eat with a spoon—it's a drink that is similar to eggnog, except it's usually served without alcohol. I was happy to create this keto version because my dad still loves boiled custard.

5 large egg yolks

½ cup granular erythritol, divided

2 cups heavy whipping cream

2 cups water

2 teaspoons vanilla powder or vanilla extract (see Note)

SPECIAL EQUIPMENT:
Candy thermometer

1. In a small bowl, whisk together the egg yolks and ¼ cup of the erythritol; set aside.

2. Attach a candy thermometer to a large heavy pot. Pour in the cream and water. Turn the heat to medium and stir in the rest of the erythritol. Continue stirring until the mixture gets hot, but don't allow it to boil.

3. Take ½ cup of the liquid out of the pot and very slowly pour it into the egg yolk mixture, whisking constantly. Then slowly pour the yolk mixture into the pot, stirring continuously. The purpose of this step is to temper the eggs so that they don't curdle.

4. Continue cooking the custard over medium heat, stirring frequently, until the temperature reaches 180°F, about 20 minutes. The custard should be thick enough to coat the back of the spoon. Remove from the heat and pour through a fine-mesh strainer into a pitcher. Stir in the vanilla powder and let cool in an ice water bath. Refrigerate until ready to serve. Serve cold in 8-ounce mugs or glasses. Store leftovers in the refrigerator for up to a week.

Note:
I like to use vanilla powder in this recipe because the flavor is more intense, but you can use either the powder or the liquid extract.

NET CARBS 2.6g				
calories	fat	protein	carbs	fiber
338	34.2g	3.8g	2.6g	0g

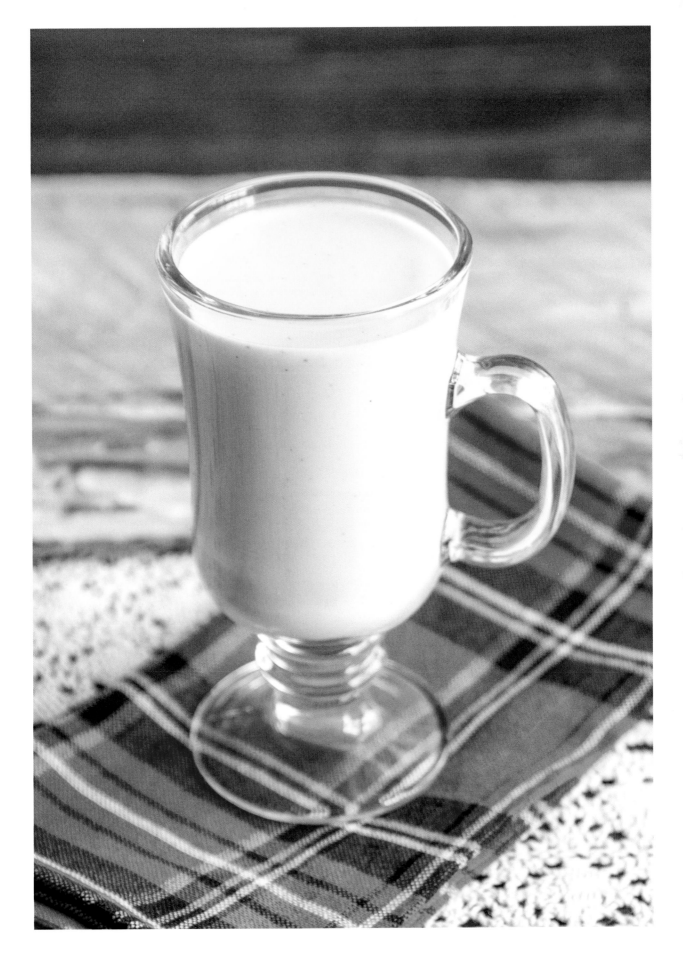

Mocha Chip Frappé

yield: 1 serving
prep time: 10 minutes

I've always loved coffee shop frappés. I liked them even before I developed a taste for regular hot coffee. Of course, those frappés are loaded with sugar and carbs! This keto version hits the spot.

1 cup strong brewed coffee, cold (see Note)

1 cup ice

2 tablespoons heavy whipping cream

2 tablespoons granular erythritol

1 tablespoon cocoa powder

1 scoop unflavored collagen peptides

1 (½-ounce) square ultra-dark chocolate (about 90% cacao), chopped

FOR SERVING (optional):

Whipped Cream (page 254)

Ultra-dark chocolate shavings (about 90% cacao)

Put all the ingredients, except the garnishes, in a blender. Blend on high speed until the frappé is smooth and frothy. Pour into a 16-ounce glass and top with whipped cream and chocolate shavings, if desired. Serve immediately.

Note:
Make sure to use a good-quality coffee that you enjoy drinking on its own. This drink is a perfect use for leftover morning coffee.

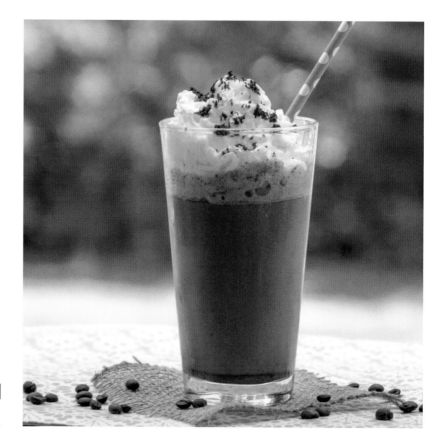

NET CARBS 4.5g				
calories	fat	protein	carbs	fiber
246	20.6g	8.9g	6g	1.5g

Frosty Keto Float

yield: 1 serving

prep time: 5 minutes, plus time to freeze mug

Root beer floats may be common in most parts of the United States, but in the South, our soda of choice for floats is Coca-Cola. How I used to love drinking a frosty Coke float loaded with ice cream! This float doesn't have ice cream or Coke in it, but the addition of real cream mimics the flavor of melted ice cream. It's delicious!

1 cup crushed ice

2 tablespoons heavy whipping cream

1 (12-ounce) can sugar-free cola or other flavored soda of choice

Liquid stevia

Whipped Cream (page 254), for serving

1. Place a 20-ounce mug in the freezer until it is frosty.

2. Place the crushed ice in the frosty mug, then pour in the cream. Slowly pour the soda over the ice and cream. Add stevia to your desired sweetness, then stir to combine. Top with whipped cream and serve immediately.

Note:

Zevia sodas are a good option for this recipe because they are sweetened with stevia. Keep a mug stored in the freezer for a frosty drink anytime you want one!

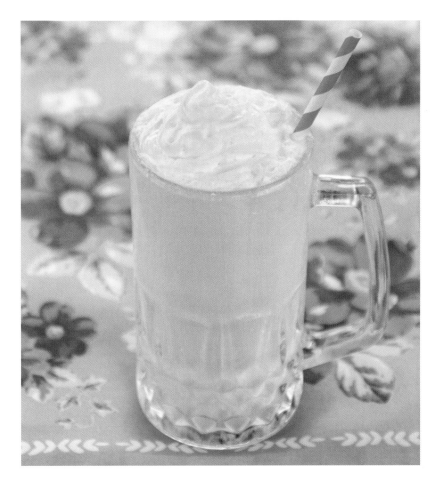

NET CARBS 0.8g				
calories	fat	protein	carbs	fiber
110	11.4g	0.6g	0.8g	0g

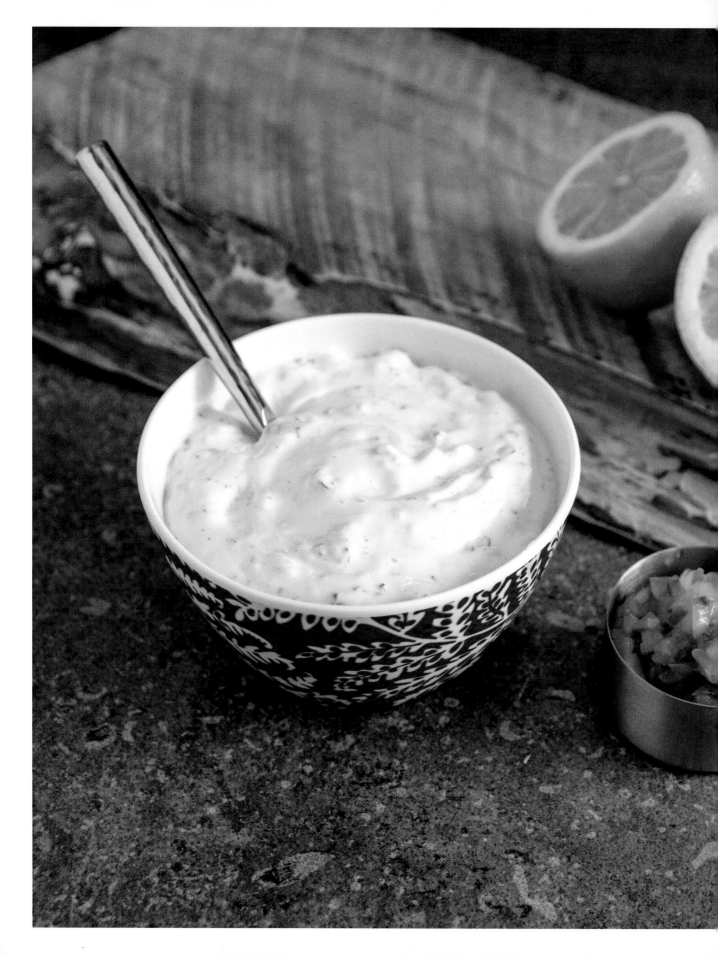

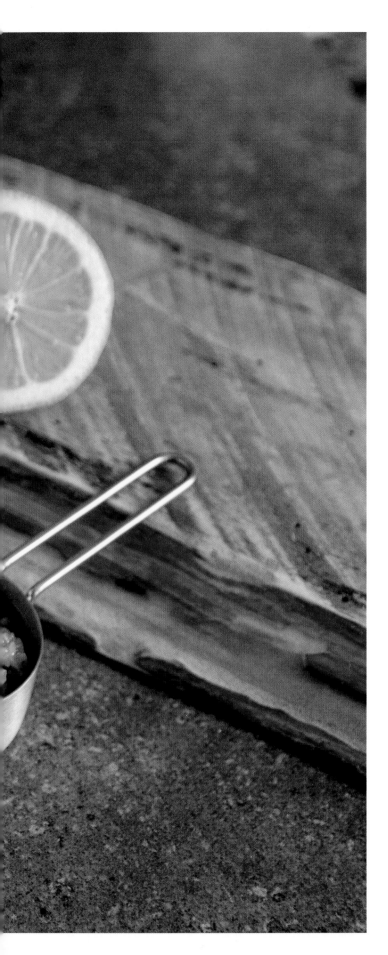

Condiments

Creole Seasoning

*yield: about ½ cup
(1 tablespoon per serving)*

prep time: 5 minutes

Make your own Creole seasoning without all those additives and sugar. You can turn down the heat by decreasing the amount of cayenne pepper, but I don't know why you'd want to! This seasoning can be used in anything you'd like to add a little kick to: eggs, meats, vegetables, or salads.

2 tablespoons paprika

2 tablespoons salt

2 tablespoons ground black pepper

1 tablespoon onion powder

1 teaspoon dried basil

1 teaspoon dried ground oregano

1 teaspoon cayenne pepper

In a small bowl, stir the ingredients together until well combined. Store in a jar with a lid. Shake before use.

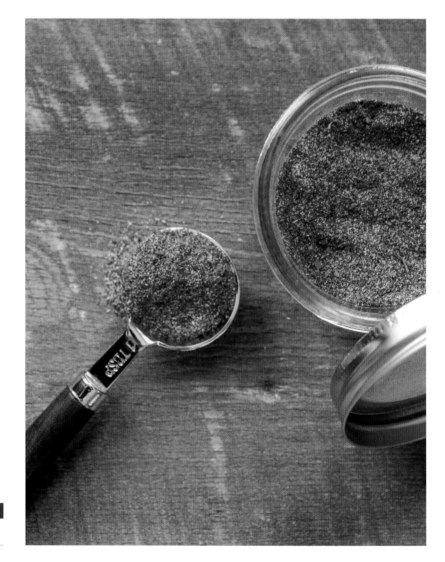

NET CARBS 1.6g				
calories	fat	protein	carbs	fiber
13	0.3g	0.5g	2.9g	1.3g

Taco Seasoning

yield: about ½ cup
(1 tablespoon per serving)
prep time: 5 minutes

This is probably my most frequently used homemade seasoning mix. For years, I used those little packets, which are loaded with additives. I'm so glad I started making my own instead! We love taco salad and eat it often.

¼ cup chili powder

2 tablespoons ground cumin

1 tablespoon smoked paprika

2 teaspoons salt

1 teaspoon ground black pepper

1 teaspoon garlic powder

1 teaspoon onion powder

1 teaspoon dried oregano leaves

In a small bowl, stir the ingredients together until well combined. Store in a jar with a lid. Shake before use.

Note:
Use 2 tablespoons of taco seasoning per pound of meat.

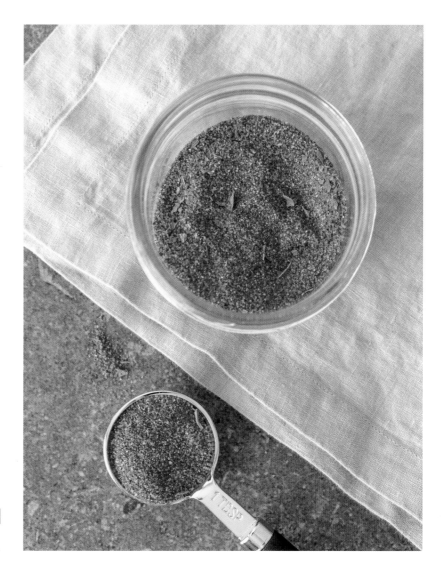

NET CARBS 2.1g				
calories	fat	protein	carbs	fiber
22	1g	1g	3.9g	2.1g

Tennessee Dry Rub

yield: about ¼ cup
prep time: 5 minutes

This dry rub is the perfect combination of smoky and spicy with a hint of sweetness. If you don't like heat, you can leave out the cayenne pepper. This blend is great on all cuts of pork. My husband likes to put it on chicken wings and even shrimp!

2 tablespoons brown sugar substitute

1 tablespoon smoked paprika

2 teaspoons ground black pepper

1 teaspoon ground cumin

1 teaspoon dried ground oregano

1 teaspoon salt

½ teaspoon onion powder

¼ teaspoon cayenne pepper

In a small bowl, stir the ingredients together until well combined. Store in a jar with a lid. Shake before use.

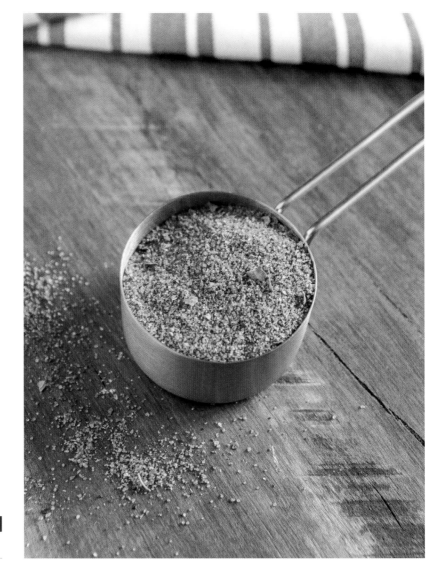

NET CARBS 6.1g				
calories	fat	protein	carbs	fiber
65	2.4g	3g	13g	6.8g

Ranch Seasoning

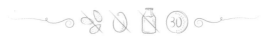

yield: about 1 cup (1 tablespoon per serving)

prep time: 5 minutes

5 tablespoons dried parsley leaves

3 tablespoons dried dill weed

2 tablespoons dried chives

2 tablespoons garlic powder

1 tablespoon dried minced onions

1 tablespoon onion powder

2 teaspoons salt

2 teaspoons ground black pepper

Once you make your own ranch seasoning, you'll never want to go back to store-bought. And it's easier to make than you might think!

In a small bowl, stir the ingredients together until well combined. Store in a jar with a lid. Shake before use.

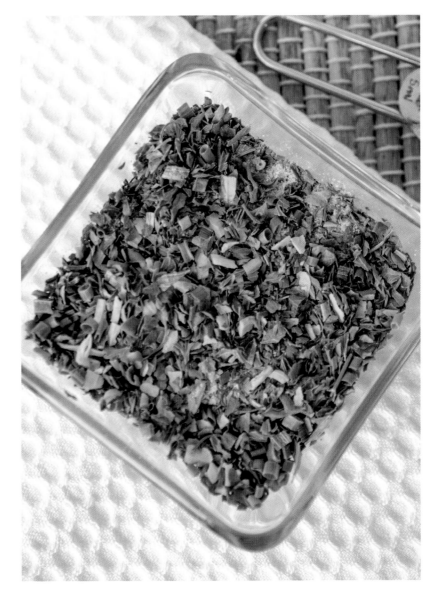

NET CARBS 1.6g				
calories	fat	protein	carbs	fiber
9	0.1g	0.5g	2g	0.4g

Ranch Dressing

*yield: about 2 cups
(¼ cup per serving)*

prep time: 5 minutes

1 cup sour cream

½ cup mayonnaise

¼ cup heavy whipping cream, plus extra if needed

1 teaspoon freshly squeezed lemon juice

2 tablespoons Ranch Seasoning (page 273)

Everyone needs a good recipe for ranch dressing! This one is delicious and easy to make, and you can feel good knowing you've avoided the added chemicals and preservatives found in most store-bought brands. Try it with the Crispy Chicken Wings!

In a small bowl, stir the ingredients together until completely blended. If the dressing is too thick, thin it with more cream, adding 1 teaspoon at a time. Store in an airtight container in the refrigerator for up to a week.

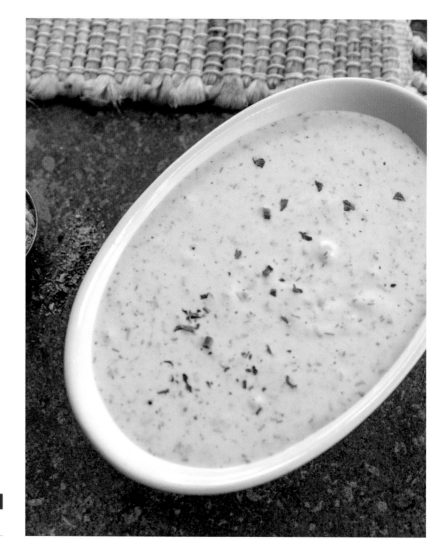

NET CARBS 0.9g				
calories	fat	protein	carbs	fiber
148	15.4g	0.6g	1g	0.1g

Buffalo Sauce

yield: about 1½ cups
(¼ cup per serving)
prep time: 5 minutes
cook time: 5 minutes

½ cup (1 stick) salted butter

1 cup Frank's RedHot sauce, room temperature

Ground black pepper

Note:
When making this recipe, it's important to use room-temperature hot sauce so that the ingredients blend well.

This sauce tastes exactly like my family's favorite restaurant Buffalo sauce. I like to serve it on shrimp. You'll find yourself wanting to put it on everything!

Melt the butter in a small saucepan over medium-low heat. Stir in the hot sauce. Stir continuously until the butter and hot sauce are completely combined. Season with pepper to taste. Remove from the heat and allow to cool for 10 minutes before serving. Store in an airtight container in the refrigerator for up to 2 weeks. Stir before using.

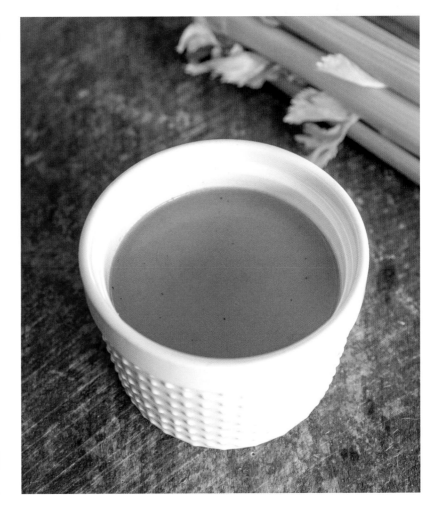

NET CARBS 0g				
calories	fat	protein	carbs	fiber
136	15.3g	0.2g	0g	0g

Tartar Sauce

yield: about 1 cup
(2 tablespoons per serving)

prep time: 10 minutes, plus
1 hour to chill

1 cup mayonnaise

¼ cup dill relish

1 tablespoon freshly
squeezed lemon juice

½ teaspoon Worcestershire
sauce

1 tablespoon dried parsley
leaves

1 teaspoon dried minced
onions

Salt and ground black
pepper, to taste

*You can't have a good fish fry without tartar sauce! A lot
of store brands contain so many unnecessary additives and
sugar. This keto-friendly version is a breeze to mix up.*

Put all the ingredients in a small bowl and stir until well
blended. Refrigerate for 1 hour before serving. Store in an
airtight container in the refrigerator for up to 5 days.

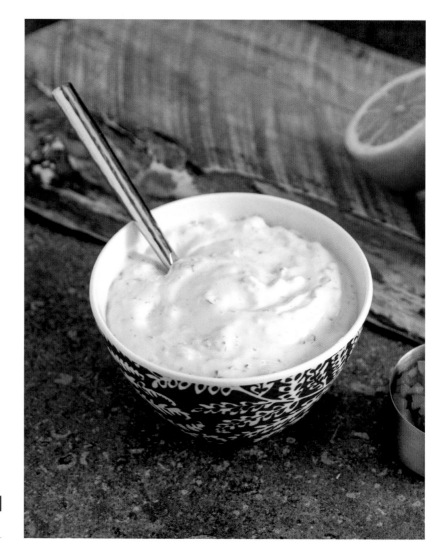

NET CARBS 0.2g				
calories	fat	protein	carbs	fiber
204	22.3g	0.1g	0.3g	0.1g

Easy BBQ Sauce

*yield: about 2 cups
(¼ cup per serving)
prep time: 5 minutes
cook time: 15 minutes*

You don't have to miss BBQ sauce! This version is perfectly delicious, and it's keto. It's a little thicker than most barbecue sauces, which makes it great to use on Barbecue Chicken Drumsticks (page 174); it can be thinned with a bit more water to suit your tastes without affecting the flavor. It is also great served alongside Slow Cooker Pulled Pork (page 158).

1 cup tomato paste

1 cup water

½ cup granular erythritol

⅓ cup apple cider vinegar

2 tablespoons Worcestershire sauce

2 teaspoons chili powder

1 teaspoon smoked paprika

½ teaspoon garlic powder

½ teaspoon ground cinnamon

½ teaspoon salt

Place all the ingredients in a medium-sized saucepan. Bring to a simmer over medium heat, then continue to simmer, stirring occasionally, for 10 to 15 minutes. Remove from the heat and allow to cool before serving. Store in an airtight container in the refrigerator for up to a week.

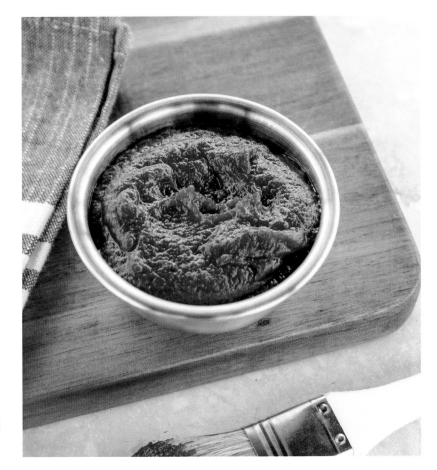

NET CARBS 3g				
calories	fat	protein	carbs	fiber
30	0.1g	1.5g	5.4g	2.4g

❧ In Appreciation ❧

Instagram and online communities—Thank you to my wonderful ketofam! I appreciate each of you for sharing this journey with me. Without you, none of this would be possible. You inspire and encourage me daily! Thank you to Dawn for being a wonderful friend and for visiting us in Tennessee!

Victory Belt Publishing—Thank you to the entire Victory Belt team for your tireless efforts to bring this dream to life. You are like family to me now. Thank you, Erich, for always being available for questions and for your great advice. The cover shoot day was an amazing day. Thank you, Lance, for being the first person to talk to me about this book. Your excitement for a Southern-themed keto cookbook encouraged me, and I enjoyed our talks about our home state of Kentucky! Thank you, Holly and Pam, for your editing and wonderful attention to detail. I learned so much from each of you! Susan, you are an amazing encourager. I'm thankful for you and our talks! Thank you to the talented design team for your beautiful work!

My husband—My recipe taste-tester. I have so much appreciation for you that it's hard to know where to start. You are my best friend and biggest supporter in life. You've been there for me in sickness and in health. Thank you for loving me unconditionally even when I didn't love myself. Thank you for believing in me and encouraging me to push on when this process got hard. I love you with all of my heart. Like you used to say back when we were dating, "Let's grow old together."

My daughter and son—Thank you for supporting your mom's crazy ideas and always being willing to try the recipes and give honest feedback. You two bring me so much joy and are my greatest blessings in life. I'm so incredibly proud of the young adults you are becoming! I'm sorry I didn't always model the greatest confidence in myself when you were growing up, but I do hope that the work I've done to turn things around will help strengthen your belief in yourselves and your resolve to chase your dreams and never give up! I love you, believe in you, and will always support and encourage you.

Dad and Mom—Thank you for being absolutely amazing parents and grandparents. You gave me such a wonderful and loving childhood. I am so blessed! Thank you for the spiritual role models you've been for me all of my life. You both inspire me daily. I could not have done this without your continued emotional support and prayers! I love you!

Family and friends—When I count my blessings, so many people come to mind—too many to name. I am thankful to each one of you who has touched my life along the way.

Kim and Machelle—My cousins, but always more like sisters, and my best friends! I love you, and I'm so blessed to have had your encouragement

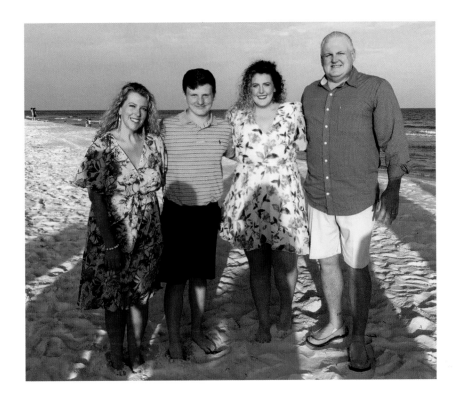

all of my life! Kim, thank you for believing in me and encouraging me to continue sharing my journey publicly and help others even when it became uncomfortable. Machelle, thank you for seeing me in a better light than I could see myself when we were teenagers and I was struggling. You both inspire in the way you live your lives—more than you'll ever know!

Cherrish—Thank you so much for allowing me to use your beautiful kitchen for the photo shoot! It was a fun and special day, and I'm thankful for the time we spent together. I love you, and I'm so proud of you!

Lisa—Although we met later in life, you are one of the best friends I've ever had! We love your family. Thank you so much for being there for me so many times when I was sick. You are one of the most humble and thoughtful people I have ever met. Thank you for all of your encouragement and recipe taste-testing while I was writing this book!

Wendy and Dorinda—Thank you for being my lifelong best friends and always loving me unconditionally. We don't get to spend nearly enough time together, but you are always in my heart!

Bill Staley and Hayley Mason—Thank you so much for the beautiful cover shot. You were so thoughtful about the details and bringing my ideas to life. I enjoyed working with you!

Chloe—I'm so glad that you did my photo shoot! I have never been comfortable getting my picture taken. Thank you for helping me feel at ease and making the process enjoyable!

Testimonials

Here are a few testimonials from people I know. The best part is that their success on the ketogenic diet isn't just about a number on a scale!

I want to begin by saying how super proud I am of Tasha and her success with the ketogenic diet. Tasha is my cousin but has been more like my sister my entire life! We grew up together. She is one of the most humble people I have ever met. As kids, I knew Tasha struggled with her weight, but her infectious personality and love for others camouflaged that fact. So I never looked at her as being overweight.

About three years ago, I found out about her keto Instagram page. It's funny now but definitely wasn't at the time. We have always told each other everything, and even though I knew she was losing weight and keeping it off this time, I really hadn't asked her for details about what it was. She just mentioned in a nonchalant way that she had this Instagram page that she hadn't really told a lot of her family/friends about. When I looked it up, I found that she had 12,000 followers! I could not believe she hadn't told me about this! We laugh now because I was really mad about it. I mean, how awesome is that, and why in the world would you not share it with everyone you knew, right? Well, the fact is, she was sharing with thousands of people, just not the ones who had been a witness to her struggle or the ones she felt would judge her. But, in fact, these are the ones who are most inspired by her! So this was the beginning of my own keto journey.

I am 45 years old and a registered nurse. I have always been really good about exercising, and I would say I am a self-motivator, except when it comes to healthy eating. I have needed to lose 10 to 15 pounds for a few years now but would find myself hungry on diets, and then I would cave in and eat. With the ketogenic diet, I was not hungry, and I was losing weight! I didn't think about my next meal as I was eating my current one. My energy level skyrocketed, and I felt in total control of my diet for the first time in a long time. Tasha has taught me simple recipes that curb my sweet tooth and fill me up. I am so excited about having this cookbook on hand!

I have several friends and coworkers who have had great success with this diet as well. I don't even call it a "diet" anymore. This is my lifestyle most of the time. I have learned that I can eat, be full, and be happy without all of those carbs.

Good luck on this journey! It's been great to me.

—Kim Carter

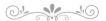

I've followed a ketogenic way of eating since November 2014. It all started when my daughter, Paige, was 17 and was diagnosed with insulin resistance. Her doctor told her to eat a ketogenic diet to keep it under control and halt its progression into possible diabetes. Neither one of us had ever heard of a ketogenic diet. We listened to the doctor with astonished looks on our faces as he told us everything she could not eat. We felt it was impossible.

After researching ketosis, it seemed pretty overwhelming and difficult, especially for a teenager! Because of that, I decided to do the diet along with her to support her and help her navigate it. Together, we learned recipes and figured out how to eat in restaurants and what to buy in the grocery store. The beginning was pretty rough for both of us, and I never thought I could make it through the holidays, let alone sustain it long term. Never eat bread or sugar? Pasta or fruit? Because we were doing it together, we supported each other and made it through. It was a terrific bonding experience with such positive results. We both lost weight and felt great. I am forever grateful to Paige's doctor for introducing this way of eating to us. Because of him, I will always eat a low-carb diet because of the way it makes me look and feel. I never would have believed that!

I lost the majority of my weight in the first two years and stalled for an entire year before buckling down and reaching goal weight in early 2018. I have lost 93 pounds (235 to 142) and seven clothing sizes (20 to 4/6), but I have also gained so much from this way of eating! After over 20 years of being on oral medication for various health problems (high blood pressure, GERD, PVCs, anemia), I am completely off all oral medications! My joints no longer ache from inflammation. My feet don't tingle. My hips don't scream in pain. I went through menopause with barely a symptom. Additionally, I began exercising in February 2018 and met my goal of running my first 5K in April. I look years younger, and I have gained the confidence to do things I never dreamed of. All from keto!

I love the ketogenic way of eating so much that I have ketoed on every vacation I have taken for the past four years. This year, that meant no pasta, pizza, or gelato in Italy. No pastries or fries in France. No bread or rice in Spain. But it also meant I felt my best and had the energy to walk up to 12 miles a day! I would not have it any other way. Eating off plan holds no appeal to me when being in ketosis feels so great!

I am so passionate about the ketogenic diet. It has helped me regain my health and my confidence, and I've made some wonderful friends along the way through Instagram! That has been one of the best resources I have ever found. The warmth of that community was instrumental in keeping me motivated and helped me to not give up. I have met people from all over the world, and they have enriched my life. I will forever be grateful that Tasha was one of them. Tasha and I first met on Instagram years ago, and we bonded over our passion for health and the ketogenic way of eating.

Let's all take time to celebrate ourselves for the choices we are making to improve our health. Don't give up! You got this! Just keep swimming!

—Dawn Marsala Delaney

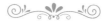

I love food. I am not a picky eater. I sort of wish I was a little picky, but I love most things and will try just about anything that's put in front of me. That being said, I didn't grow up having weight issues and ate what I thought was a pretty healthy diet. Like most people, as you age, food choices become even more important for health/weight. Several years ago, I started eating low-carb, not super strict, but I definitely was cutting out typical high-carb items like bread, rice, and pasta. I did it mainly to lose a few pounds, again nothing major—maybe 10 pounds or so. I lost that weight and slowly started to eat some carb-heavy foods again. I don't weigh myself, but I know my clothes were fitting a little more snugly. My dear friend Tasha had been eating strictly keto for a while, and she would always pass on tips and great recipes. I had been thinking about going really strict and eating only keto; I just needed to commit to it. Since I hadn't grown up with weight issues, I also hadn't yo-yo'd with different diets, and I was never into trying the latest and greatest diet fads. One area I struggled with was dessert. I LOVE DESSERT. Tasha mentioned that eating keto actually helped with these cravings because eating keto cuts your sugar intake. I think it was timing. I had been thinking about trying keto, and then, when Tasha mentioned the reduced sugar craving, that sold me. Well, that and all of the amazing and easy meals Tasha would make. I don't love cooking, and I love choices, so this was perfect.

I have been eating keto for almost a year and a half straight. I have lost over 20 pounds. The weight loss has been great, but knowing that I am cutting my sugar is my favorite part, because cutting sugar is *so* hard! My family sometimes eats keto and sometimes doesn't. It's a choice I made, and I will find a way to make it work whether I'm at home, on the run, or at my favorite restaurant. It's really not even a thought at this point. There are just too many delicious, easy, and cheap ways that make eating keto a no-brainer.

—Lisa Presnell

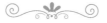

My husband and I had some success with the Atkins Diet in 2002. We both lost quite a bit of weight. We were in our thirties then. Of course, we failed to stay committed due to busy lives and limited dietary options.

Fast-forward to 2017. We both decided it was time to get healthy. It wasn't just about weight loss or diet. Becoming healthy meant not only getting active again, but also changing our eating habits to help us lose weight and feel good. Having had some previous success with low-carb, we decided this would be our choice. Dr. Chris Newton, our chiropractor, told us about Tasha's Instagram page. Her recipes and ideas have truly changed our lives!

Tasha made it easy to stick to the keto diet. She gave great advice not only about snacking and eating out (including how to order keto at specific restaurants), but also how to make our favorite foods keto-friendly. We have eaten pizza, tacos, cakes, cookies, etc., and with Tasha's guidance, these were all keto-friendly!

This sweet lady has made the difference in our lives and our health. Through exercise and the keto diet, my husband lost 95 pounds and I lost 25. But more importantly, we are active again. We feel better. And our health is much improved. We can't thank Tasha enough for her contribution to our success. I am so glad to have so many wonderful keto-friendly recipes in one place with this new book!

Fans for life!

—Rebecca Foster

Measurement and Cooking Conversion Tables

For those who live outside the United States and use metric measurements.

LIQUIDS

¼ teaspoon	1.25 ml
½ teaspoon	2.5 ml
1 teaspoon	5 ml
1 tablespoon	15 ml
¼ cup	60 ml
⅓ cup	80 ml
½ cup	125 ml
1 cup	250 ml

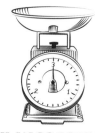

DRY INGREDIENTS

1 oz	28 g
2 oz	55 g
3 oz	85 g
4 oz	115 g
8 oz	225 g
12 oz	340 g
16 oz / 1 pound	455 g
32 oz	907 g

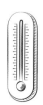

TEMPERATURE

275°F	140°C
300°F	150°C
325°F	170°C
350°F	180°C
375°F	190°C
400°F	200°C
425°F	220°C
450°F	230°C

❧ Resources ❧

A few of my favorite products

It's exciting to see a growing number of companies offering convenience foods that make the keto life easier. Due to the popularity of low-carb diets, I expect this number to keep increasing. Here are just a few of the products that I use. You should always research new products and the ingredients they contain to make sure that they are right for you. I have listed the company websites so that you can read more about their offerings, but I recommend doing a Google search to find the best prices.

ALTERNASWEETS
www.alternasweets.com
Stevia-sweetened ketchup and barbecue sauce.

CHOSEN FOODS
chosenfoods.com
Mayonnaise made with avocado oil.

GOOD DEE'S
www.gooddees.com
Yummy low-carb and gluten-free baking mixes for brownies, cakes, cookies, and pancakes.

KERRYGOLD
www.kerrygoldusa.com
Delicious grass-fed butter. You do not have to use grass-fed butter on keto, but I recommend this brand because it tastes better than any other store-bought butter I've tried. Kerrygold also makes a variety of cheeses; the Dubliner is my favorite.

LAKANTO
www.lakanto.com
A variety of monk fruit–sweetened products. I sometimes use their granular sweetener, which is a blend of monk fruit and erythritol. Lakanto also makes sugar-free maple-flavored syrup.

LILY'S
lilyssweets.com
I use Lily's stevia-sweetened chocolate chips for baking and enjoy their chocolate bars for snacking—they're delicious!

MOON CHEESE
mooncheese.com
Crunchy cheese snacks. My favorite flavors are Pepper Jack and Cheddar, but I'm also enjoying the newest flavor, Sriracha.

PERFECT KETO
www.perfectketo.com
A variety of supplements. I often use their collagen peptides and MCT oil. They make a great MCT oil powder, which is my favorite form of MCT oil because of how well it blends and digests. It also comes in a variety of flavors.

PRIMAL PALATE

www.primalpalate.com

Organic spices and spice blends, with lots of no-sugar-added options. The taco seasoning is amazing. Primal Palate also offers seasoning packets in flavors such as French Onion and Garden Ranch.

SUKRIN GOLD

sukrinusa.com

I like Sukrin's brown sugar alternative and use it in any recipe that calls for brown sugar.

WHISPS

www.whisps.com

Parmesan cheese crisps that come in a variety of flavors. They are great for snacking, but I also like using them as a salad topper.

ZEVIA

www.zevia.com

Stevia-sweetened sodas. They come in a wide variety of flavors and can be found at most health food stores.

Books and websites

Here are just a few good resources to get you started. I encourage you to do your own online search because there are many more books, websites, and other resources that wonderfully represent the ketogenic lifestyle.

BOOKS

The Art and Science of Low Carb Living, by Stephen D. Phinney and Jeff S. Volek

The Case Against Sugar, by Gary Taubes

The Complete Guide to Fasting, by Jason Fung, MD, and Jimmy Moore

Keto Clarity, by Jimmy Moore and Eric C. Westman, MD

WEBSITES

alldayidreamaboutfood.com

dietdoctor.com

grassfedgirl.com

healthfulpursuit.com

ketogenicgirl.com

mariamindbodyhealth.com

peaceloveandlowcarb.com

sugarfreemom.com

thecastawaykitchen.com

Recipe Quick Reference

RECIPE	PAGE	🌿	🚫	🧂	30
Smoked Sausage and Mushroom Breakfast Skillet	56	✓			
Cowboy Breakfast Skillet	58	✓			
Grain-Free Granola	60				
Skillet Pancake Puff	62	✓			✓
Waffles	64	✓			
Egg Muffins	66	✓			
Home-Fried Bacon Radishes	68	✓	✓	✓	
Sausage Gravy	70	O	✓		✓
Drop Biscuits	72				✓
Skillet Cornbread	74				
Cinnamon Muffins	76				✓
Blueberry Muffins	78				
Lemon Poppy Seed Loaf	80	✓			
Zucchini Bread	82				
Artichoke Dip	86	✓			
Cheesy Sausage Balls	88		✓		
Pimento Cheese	90	✓			
Dill Pickle Chips	92	✓			✓
Cheese Crisps	94	✓	✓		✓
Sweet Pepper Poppers	96	✓	✓		✓
Hushpuppies	98				✓
Deviled Eggs	100	✓		✓	
Pecan Ranch Cheese Ball	102		✓		
Pulled Pork Buffalo Dip for Two	104	✓	✓		✓
Cucumber Finger Sandwiches	106	✓	✓		✓
Baked BLT Dip	108	✓			
Bacon-Stuffed Mushrooms	110	✓	✓		
Broccoli Cheese Soup	114	✓	✓		✓
Loaded Fauxtato Soup	116	✓	✓		✓
Taco Soup	118	✓	✓		
Cheeseburger Soup	120	✓	✓		
Tomato Basil Soup	122	✓	✓		
Easy Chili	124	✓	✓	✓	
Gumbo	126		✓		
Tuna Salad-Stuffed Peppers	128	✓		✓	✓
Classic Egg Salad	130	✓		✓	✓
Broccoli Cauliflower Salad	132	✓			
Creamy Coleslaw	134	✓		✓	

RECIPE	PAGE	🌱	🚫	🍶	30
Southern Fauxtato Salad	136	✓		✓	
BLT Wedge Salad	138	✓	✓		✓
Marinated Cucumber Salad	140	✓	✓	✓	
Easy Chicken Salad	142	✓		✓	
Cornbread Salad	144				
Spinach Salad with Hot Bacon Dressing	146			✓	✓
Open-Faced Sloppy Joes	150	✓	✓	✓	
Memphis-Style Ribs	152	✓	✓	✓	
Shrimp Creole	154	✓	✓		
Chili Cheese Pot Pie	156				
Slow Cooker Pulled Pork	158	✓	✓	✓	
Crispy Chicken Wings	160	✓	✓	✓	
Cheeseburger "Mac" Helper	162	✓	✓		✓
Creamy Broccoli and Ground Beef Casserole	164	✓	✓		
Bacon Cheeseburger Mini Meatloaves	166	✓			
Sheet Pan Garlic Butter Shrimp	168	✓	✓		✓
Ground Beef Stroganoff	170	✓	✓		✓
Southern Fish Fry	172	✓			
Barbecue Chicken Drumsticks	174	✓	✓	✓	
Reverse Sear Garlic Rosemary Rib-Eye Steaks	176	✓	✓		
Cajun Sausage and Rice	178	✓	✓	✓	
Slow Cooker Bourbon Chicken	180	✓	✓	✓	
Fried Chicken	182	✓			
Barbecue Pulled Pork Pizza	184				
Salmon Patties	186				
Pizza-Stuffed Peppers	188	✓	✓		
Butter Roasted Turkey	190				
Fried Cabbage and Bacon	194	✓	✓	✓	✓
Green Bean Bacon Bundles	196	✓	✓	✓	
Loaded Roasted Cauliflower	198	✓	✓		
Hash Brown Casserole	200	✓	✓		
Easy Cheesy Caulirice	202	✓	✓		✓
Roasted Spaghetti Squash	204	✓	✓	✓	
Turnip Fries with Dipping Sauce	206	✓			
Sausage Cornbread Dressing	208				
Easy Caulimash	210	✓	✓		✓
Parmesan Asparagus	211	✓	✓		
Garlic Butter Roasted Radishes	212	✓	✓		

RECIPE	PAGE	✿	◯	🥛	30
Bacon Roasted Cabbage Steaks	213	✓	✓	✓	✓
Old-Fashioned Green Beans	214	✓	✓		
Blistered Okra	216	✓	✓		✓
Fried Green Tomatoes	218	✓			
Keto Cheesecake with Pecan Almond Crust	222				
Peanut Butter Chocolate Chip Cookie Bars	224			✓	✓
Fruit Pizza	226				
Peanut Butter Pie Bites with Chocolate Drizzle	228		✓		
Chocolate Pecan Pie	230				
Praline Toasted Pecans	232		✓		✓
One-Bowl Butter Cookies	234				✓
Strawberry Shortcakes	236				✓
Quick Blackberry Cobbler for Two	238		✓		✓
Easy Truffles	240	O	✓		
Kentucky Bourbon Balls	242		✓		
Chocolate Pudding	244	O	✓		
Dark Chocolate Coconut Fat Bombs	246	✓	✓		
Glazed Coconut Bundt Cake	248				
Pumpkin Pie	250				
Almond Flour Crust	252		✓		
Whipped Cream	254	✓	✓		✓
Strawberry Milkshake	258		✓		✓
Keto Berry Smoothie	259		✓	✓	✓
Keto Sweet Tea	260	✓	✓	✓	
Hot Chocolate	261		✓		✓
Lemonade for One	262	✓	✓	✓	✓
Bulletproof Coffee	263	✓	✓		✓
Southern Boiled Custard	264	✓			
Mocha Chip Frappé	266	✓	✓		✓
Frosty Keto Float	267	✓	✓		
Creole Seasoning	270	✓	✓	✓	✓
Taco Seasoning	271	✓	✓	✓	✓
Tennessee Dry Rub	272	✓	✓	✓	✓
Ranch Seasoning	273	✓	✓	✓	✓
Ranch Dressing	274	✓			✓
Buffalo Sauce	275	✓	✓		✓
Tartar Sauce	276	✓		✓	
Easy BBQ Sauce	277	✓	✓	✓	✓

Recipe Index

Breakfast & Breads

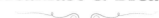

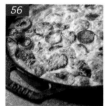
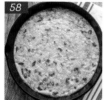
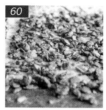
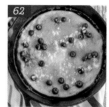
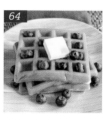
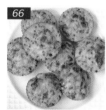
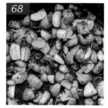
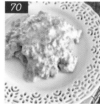
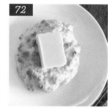
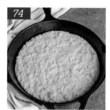
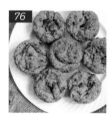
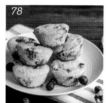
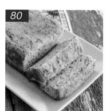
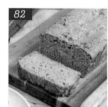

Appetizers & Snacks

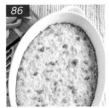
Artichoke Dip

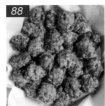
Cheesy
Sausage Balls

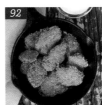
Pimento Cheese

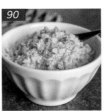
Dill Pickle Chips

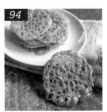
Cheese Crisps

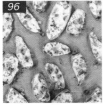
Sweet Pepper
Poppers

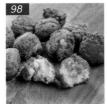
Hushpuppies

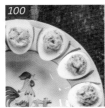
Deviled Eggs

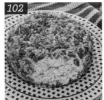
Pecan Ranch
Cheese Ball

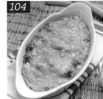
Pulled Pork
Buffalo Dip
for Two

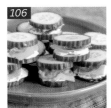
Cucumber Finger
Sandwiches

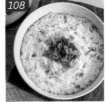
Baked BLT Dip

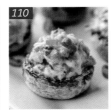
Bacon-Stuffed
Mushrooms

Soups & Salads

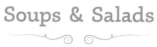

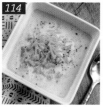
114
Broccoli Cheese
Soup

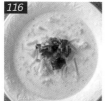
116
Loaded Fauxtato
Soup

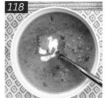
118
Taco Soup

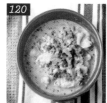
120
Cheeseburger
Soup

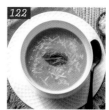
122
Tomato Basil Soup

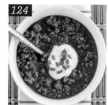
124
Easy Chili

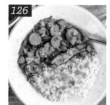
126
Gumbo

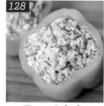
128
Tuna Salad-
Stuffed Peppers

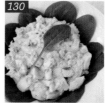
130
Classic Egg Salad

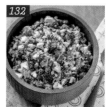
132
Broccoli
Cauliflower Salad

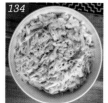
134
Creamy Coleslaw

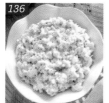
136
Southern Fauxtato
Salad

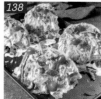
138
BLT Wedge Salad

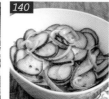
140
Marinated
Cucumber Salad

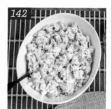
142
Easy Chicken
Salad

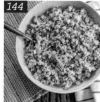
144
Cornbread Salad

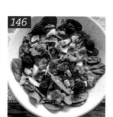
146
Spinach Salad
with Hot Bacon
Dressing

Main Dishes

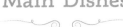

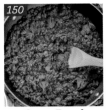
Open-Faced
Sloppy Joes

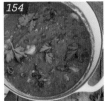
Memphis-Style
Ribs

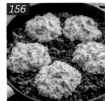
Shrimp Creole

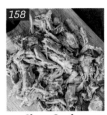
Chili Cheese
Pot Pie

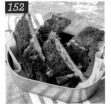
Slow Cooker
Pulled Pork

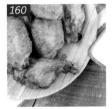
Crispy
Chicken Wings

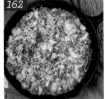
Cheeseburger
"Mac" Helper

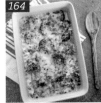
Creamy Broccoli
and
Ground Beef
Casserole

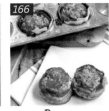
Bacon
Cheeseburger
Mini Meatloaves

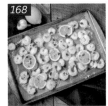
Sheet Pan
Garlic Butter
Shrimp

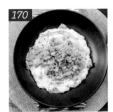
Ground Beef
Stroganoff

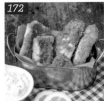
Southern Fish Fry

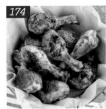
Barbecue Chicken
Drumsticks

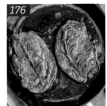
Reverse Sear
Garlic Rosemary
Rib-Eye Steaks

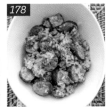
Cajun Sausage
and Rice

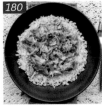
Slow Cooker
Bourbon Chicken

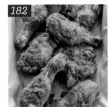
Fried Chicken

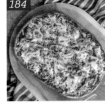
Barbecue
Pulled Pork Pizza

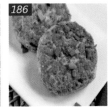
Salmon Patties

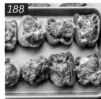
Pizza-Stuffed
Peppers

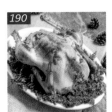
Butter Roasted
Turkey

Side Dishes

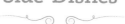

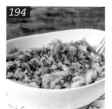
194
Fried Cabbage
and Bacon

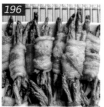
196
Green Bean
Bacon Bundles

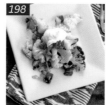
198
Loaded Roasted
Cauliflower

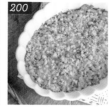
200
Hash Brown
Casserole

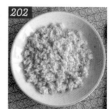
202
Easy Cheesy
Caulirice

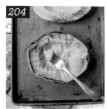
204
Roasted
Spaghetti Squash

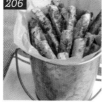
206
Turnip Fries with
Dipping Sauce

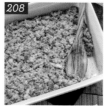
208
Sausage Cornbread
Dressing

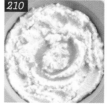
210
Easy Caulimash

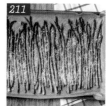
211
Parmesan
Asparagus

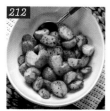
212
Garlic Butter
Roasted Radishes

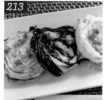
213
Bacon Roasted
Cabbage Steaks

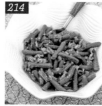
214
Old-Fashioned
Green Beans

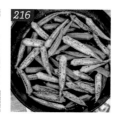
216
Blistered Okra

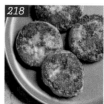
218
Fried Green
Tomatoes

Desserts

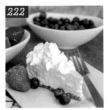
Keto Cheesecake
with Pecan
Almond Crust

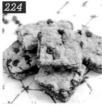
Peanut Butter
Chocolate Chip
Cookie Bars

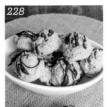
Fruit Pizza

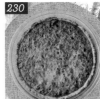
Peanut Butter
Pie Bites with
Chocolate Drizzle

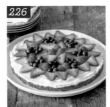
Chocolate Pecan
Pie

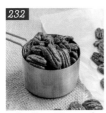
Praline Toasted
Pecans

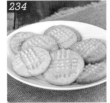
One-Bowl
Butter Cookies

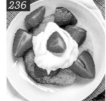
Strawberry
Shortcakes

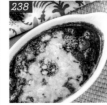
Quick Blackberry
Cobbler for Two

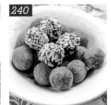
Easy Truffles

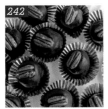
Kentucky
Bourbon Balls

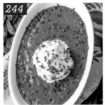
Chocolate Pudding

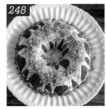
Dark Chocolate
Coconut
Fat Bombs

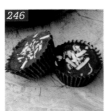
Glazed Coconut
Bundt Cake

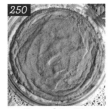
Pumpkin Pie

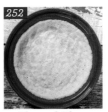
Almond Flour
Crust

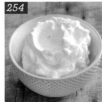
Whipped Cream

Drinks

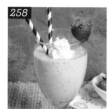
Strawberry
Milkshake

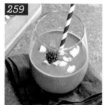
Keto Berry
Smoothie

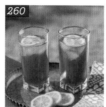
Keto Sweet Tea

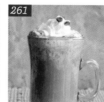
Hot Chocolate

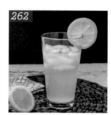
Lemonade
for One

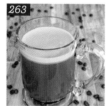
Bulletproof
Coffee

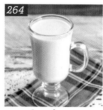
Southern
Boiled Custard

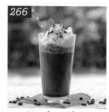
Mocha Chip
Frappé

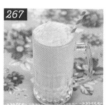
Frosty Keto Float

Condiments

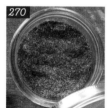
Creole Seasoning

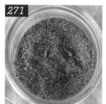
Taco Seasoning

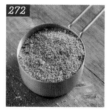
Tennessee
Dry Rub

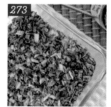
Ranch Seasoning

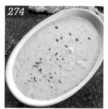
Ranch Dressing

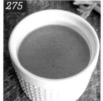
Buffalo Sauce

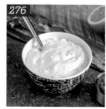
Tartar Sauce

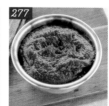
Easy BBQ Sauce

General Index